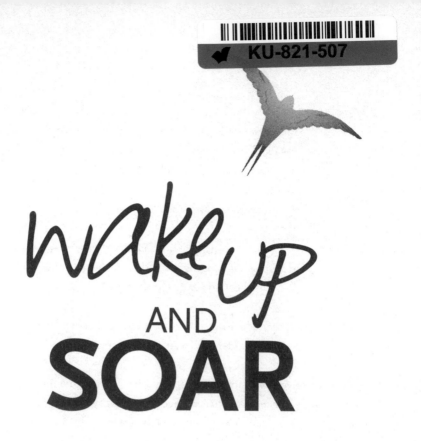

wake up
AND
SOAR

HOW TO MASTER YOUR OWN WELLBEING

CHRIS NELSON

This edition published in the UK and USA 2016 by
Watkins, an imprint of Watkins Media Limited
19 Cecil Court, London WC2N 4EZ

enquiries@watkinspublishing.com

1 3 5 7 9 10 8 6 4 2

Typeset by JCS Publishing Services Ltd, www.jcs-publishing.co.uk

Printed and bound in Finland

A CIP record for this book is available from the British Library

ISBN: 978-1-78028-914-4

www.watkinspublishing.com

Contents

Acknowledgments

I would like to thank Penny for her wise and timely prompt – *'You have a different voice from others, and it's important that you publish the book.'* I want to thank Trina for her unstinting support throughout the project. A big thank you to Jo, Carly, Deborah, Nicola, Jillian, Vicky and the whole team at Watkins for believing in me.

Thank you to my mother, father, sister, brother, nieces, nephews and friends who have co-created the life experiences which have forged the backbone of the book. My gratitude to Linda, Laura, Sian, Tobie, Charlie, Matthias and Shikha, Michael and all those at Ashiyana. Special thanks go to Satyananda, for being my spiritual guide. Lastly, and by no means least, I thank YOU for having decided to buy this book, since this breathes life into the bigger vision that I shall speak of later.

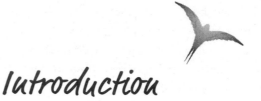

Introduction

Our modern day lifestyles are frequently out of balance, with enormous numbers of people experiencing increasing levels of stress and chronic disease. Many of us have lost our essential connection with Mother Nature, and therefore also, with our own inner nature. In the last few decades we have created a digital world that is characterized by greed, individualism, breakdown of community and our earthly biosphere is being increasingly ravaged. More than ever before, we are being called to question our purpose here on planet Earth, and the answer can often appear to be elusive.

What is the underlying reason behind our thoughts, our words, our actions and our resulting life path? What is it that fundamentally motivates and inspires us? Underneath our cultural differences, isn't there a common desire that links us all — a single thread which weaves itself through the complex fabric of life and human history?

Isn't it simply the quest to be happy, healthy and fulfilled?

Don't we all want to smile inwardly as we awaken in the morning; and not perhaps for any specific reason, but just in recognition of the fact that we are alive? Don't we all want to live our lives in a way that invites our spirit to shine brightly? Wouldn't we ideally choose to be the best that we can be? Recognizing and employing our unique gifts, yet not being limited by our shortcomings; learning to trust ourselves so that we make intelligent lifestyle choices, and spending time in supportive environments that reflect our own inner beauty.

Wake Up and SOAR offers an approach to life in this 21st Century with its bountiful possibilities and beauty, and yet equal measure of suffering. It seeks to simplify the complexity of life through using natural wisdom that has been handed down through the ages, and which today is being validated by modern science. This wisdom is present all around us in the form of Mother Nature, which has informed all of the ancient health-promoting systems.

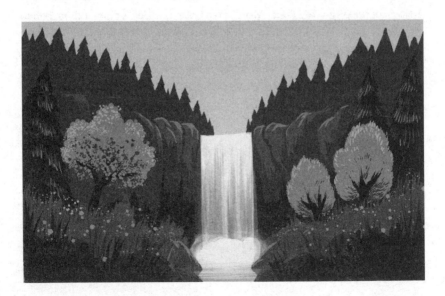

Introduction

To avail ourselves of this wisdom, we need only to slow down, breathe and observe the ways of nature. As Etty Hillesum said, 'Sometimes the most important thing in a whole day is the rest we take between two deep breaths.'

We humans are designed to flow, just like the seasons. Even our breath has a rhythm like the tide, ebbing and flowing – when we breathe in we draw in life force, or 'prana', and when we breathe out we let go of tension, tiredness and toxins. All that we truly require for life on earth is air, water, food, sun and sleep. Though to live well and embrace the full gamut of life's possibilities, we must consider what our unique purpose is here on planet Earth.

This book is a call to live your life as magnificently and fully as you possibly can. It invites you to see life as a compelling possibility which offers you your own blank canvas with which to create a masterpiece – that of your life. It is inviting you towards the ongoing awakening of your individual potential – sensing your deepest dreams, and trusting in your right to pursue those dreams so that they might light your way.

Since the dawn of time humans have been obsessed with outer space. We've reached for the stars, measuring their brightness and trajectories, seeking to explain all that we see in the night sky and the distant reaches of our fertile imagination. Rarely satisfied with the magic of nature within and surrounding us, we have forever clutched at anything that was seemingly out of our reach, as if declaring that what we already had was not enough.

Our 'outer obsession' has always been a defining element of the human experience, in spite of the fact that wise beings through the ages have urged us to look inwards, towards our own inner galaxies, stars and planetary systems. Yet outer space is in fact a wonderful guide for the journey that we so ardently avoid, since what we seek outwardly is a direct reflection of the inner sanctum of our being. The space which we crave up and out there is also to be found within us, since, as modern science has shown, the macrocosm is but a reflection of the microcosm.

There is a vast chasm of limitless spaciousness at the core of our being, which in any case is not separate from the outer space that we perceive beyond our little planet called Earth. In short, the outer human quest is nothing other than our deep desire to journey inwards back to our Source,¹ disguised as something apparently more stimulating.

Through introspection we can remember our connection with this Source. From here, all is well, and our mind-made problems melt away. From this space of inner calm, we can transcend many of our apparent limitations — our genetic predispositions, our unhealthy environments and our ego mind. We will discover that we are, and always have been, able to create our lives according to our deepest desires.

We have a great deal to learn from the way in which Mother Nature effortlessly goes about her business. Where we differ from the rest of nature perhaps, is our capacity for enjoying and suffering our ups and downs, since we are deeply emotional beings with a magnificent capacity for self-reflection. We humans therefore have the seemingly unique possibility for consciously growing and transforming.

When you slow down, observe inwardly, and accept all that is arising within and without, whilst not attaching to anything, you will naturally relax deeply. In this way you can watch your mind-made 'story' play itself out upon the private cinema screen of your inner being. Through exercising your capacity for acceptance of life, just as it is, you develop a healthy perspective on life – one that is fueled by a fresh awareness of what this moment calls for, rather than falling back on your default setting of past conditioning. You will sense the inevitable chain of events – your thoughts, words and actions, and how you are, therefore, endlessly attracting your life towards you.

Over the last couple of centuries, science has eclipsed both religion and nature. This has heralded an exceptional time in human history, where groundbreaking technological developments have been emerging at an accelerating rate. So much so, that we really have little idea of what the future looks like. There has never been such a pantheon of choice available to us, and a richness of life to explore. Yet this possibility for excessive consumption has seemingly fueled our pursuit of the superficial blip of calm and happiness which the attainment of 'outer' success yields.

Real success has little to do with reaching ever higher levels on a linear scale of money, possessions, power or or any other form of material gain. It is about depth of experience. This means simply that you stay inwardly connected whatever you are doing. The more that you live life from this deeper dimension, the happier you will be. You need to remove the shroud which masks the glow of your inner being, just as fog casts a blanket over a crystal clear lake.

When you take care of your body you invite health, and when you take care of your mind and emotions you become happy. When you are healthy and happy you feed your spirit, and have an abundance of life force which you can share with others. So, taking good care of yourself naturally causes you to want to give to others. When you give of yourself willingly, you open yourself to receiving many times in return, and your gratitude for this feeds you deeply. The happier you are, the healthier you are and the greater your life force is. This creates a virtuous circle of giving and receiving love, which causes you to love your life and feel deeply fulfilled.

There is a beautiful side effect to loving your life, which is that you cause others to transform. Therefore your own personal evolution is the key to moving the whole of humanity onto a more benign path. Not only are you the master of your own wellbeing, but you, and all of us collectively, are responsible for the future of the human race:

We are the masters of our own health and happiness and together we create the world

This book is about how *you* can capitalize upon such a compelling possibility. To do so, you must realize that life is inviting you to be the best that you can be, in every moment; and it is how you respond to this invitation that determines the trajectory of your wellbeing. Your own future, and the future of humankind, will look much like the past, until and unless we – individuals like you and me – consistently nudge human evolution in a positive direction by loving our lives.

In the words of Mahatma Gandhi – 'Be the change that you want to see in the world.' Let this change be a personal awakening to your highest possibility. Once you set forth on this path you will become a beacon of light for other adventurous souls, who also prefer to walk the path less trodden rather than amble along resigned to a life of mediocrity.

This book implores you to stop and contemplate your inner terrain. It invites you on a journey of exploration towards something deep within you – something that is calling out and asking to be recognized, and which all of us share at the Source of our being – the human spirit. It is in this recognition of the profound depth of your being, that you discover the wellspring of joy, health and happiness that man has been seeking since time immemorial.

My invitation is to slow down, relax and to not be obsessed with over-achievement and being habitually busy; to nourish your body without excess or frugality, to feed your mind without strain or ignorance, and to gently flow with life.

Who Am I?

I would like to introduce myself to you. My name is Chris. I have a passion for wellbeing, and I believe that we all have the possibility to live a deeply fulfilling life.

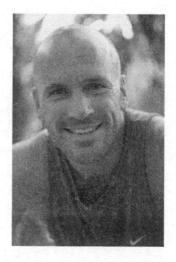

When I was 24, I created a food retail business similar to Pret A Manger. I was full of exuberance, but was also very impulsive. I had plenty of vision, but lacked business acumen. I made every single mistake that a young, inexperienced entrepreneur can make. Not surprisingly, after four and half years, during the final one of which interest rates rose from 7 per cent to 15 per cent, I went into voluntary liquidation. This was a sobering, but extremely important lesson for me.

I then spent a few years traveling around Europe involved with a sales training business, which gave me a taste for different cultures and languages, and what it was like to live in pristine nature. It was also at this time that I discovered yoga. My overriding concern was how to calm my mind, and I remember vividly the inner voice which was quietly urging me to slow down and relax. I was also increasingly aware of a dream that I'd had since my university days, which was to build a retreat center somewhere in the tropics.

I returned to London, and began to explore the world of wellbeing and holistic therapies. I also knew that I needed to make a sizable amount of money in order to realize my dream. Fortunately, I had something of a talent for property design, and having dabbled with property before, I jumped headlong into property development.

At the same time, I was attending every possible class of yoga that I could, at the 'Innergy Centre' in north-west London. The founder, Fausto, was a highly charismatic Italian who was steadfastly focused on his vision – running a little yoga sanctuary in London that taught classical Hatha yoga. It was more of an urban ashram than a yoga studio, though, and when we weren't attending or teaching the yoga classes, we hung out as a little tribe, cooking and eating, chanting and singing, and debating life's issues. Fausto, and Innergy, were a great inspiration for me.

Introduction

Amongst his many talents, Fausto had a strong intuition for when to push his students out of the nest. After four incredible years at Innergy, I was encouraged to develop my teaching experience further afield. As well as teaching at a number of yoga centers and health clubs in west and south-west London, I also created my own private classes, and a yoga retreat business. This latter activity was a key factor in my search for a little piece of paradise where I could build my own yoga center.

Having checked out many beautiful spots around the globe, I settled upon a beautiful palm grove on a river by the sea in the north of Goa, and 'Ashiyana' was born. The name was suggested to me by an Indian friend, and as she spoke the syllables – A-shi-ya-na – I knew that this was the name for my center. It sounded so beautiful and flowing. She then told me the meaning of this Sanskrit word – 'home', 'sanctuary' or 'place of rest'. It couldn't have been more perfect, since it encapsulated precisely what I wanted to create.

In the summer of 1999, a few years before this, I met Satyananda. One Saturday afternoon, together with a few friends from Innergy, I attended a small 'Satsang' gathering at the Friend's Meeting House in Ealing. For the first time in my life, I experienced someone speaking directly from their heart to my heart. From that moment on, my perspective on life shifted, and Satyananda became a key figure in my life. What I've written in this book derives from the whole of my life experience. But perhaps most of all it has been informed by my last ten years of building and nurturing Ashiyana, together with the seventeen years of being on silent retreats with Satyananda. These two influences have provided the incubator within which I've laughed, stumbled and grown, endlessly knocking my head against the walls of my life experience.

Ashiyana has been the laboratory for my experiments with yoga, alternative therapies and vast amounts of creative endeavor; Satyananda's retreats, and his friendship, have been the guiding light which has allowed me to regularly reset my internal navigation system.

In creating Ashiyana, I simply manifested my dream sanctuary, in the knowledge that others like me were probably after the same sort of 'home away from home'. The Ashiyana Retreat Village has grown into a flourishing center for urbanites seeking respite from their fast-paced, western lifestyles. Satyananda, whom I shall speak more of during the book, has been my spiritual guide, who has enabled me to realize my own Master within.

Over the last few years, I have discovered a love of writing, which has, after several attempts, resulted in this book. The impulse to write emerged without warning, and with great intensity. I remember finishing a silent retreat with Satyananda, after which I read a beautiful book about an Hawaiian healing system, and then words just started to pour out of me.

I have written a few books and short stories, none of which was published, but each served as a catalyst for something important. For example, the first book became the inspiration for the Ashiyana yoga teacher training that we run. Another book inspired me and two friends to write a film script. Let's see what happens to that. And one of the short stories is called 'Taming the Lake Monster', which you will have the chance to read in just a minute.

I tend to write about awakening, in one form or another, since I feel that this is so necessary for us humans today. By awakening, I mean remembering the Source of our being, our true nature – loving, joyful and calm. The call to awaken has always been there, but the palpable need for us to do so has perhaps never been so great. I am fascinated by the juxtaposition of challenge and opportunity that faces us in the world today: the challenge of living at a time of spiraling stress, chronic disease, inequality and wanton disregard for our earthly biosphere; juxtaposed with the incredible opportunity which this Digital Age offers us.

Over the years I've watched our guests coming over the wooden bridge at Ashiyana. I've spent time chatting with them, realizing what it is that has caused them to book a retreat or holiday with us. I have heard about their worries and concerns, and how these have manifested in their bodies as stress, chronic pain and disease. I have observed how, even over a short time, the stressors in life have increased in number and force.

The 'Hot Bath' Effect

Through this experience at Ashiyana, I have been given a bird's-eye view of what it is that creates our stress and problems at the coal-face of our western lives, as well as what it is that we can do to redress these imbalances. I have also observed that due to our human tendencies, most wellbeing experiences are subject to what I call the 'hot bath' effect. We climb into the bath and feel great, because it's hot and nurturing. But when we get out of the bath, we quickly cool down, and pretty soon the experience has worn off and is little more than a distant memory.

This obviously varies from one experience to another, and certainly there may have been books that we've read and courses that we've attended which have had a profound impact upon our being. But I still believe that in the main, there is an issue with our capacity to integrate a wellbeing experience (such as a yoga retreat, a self-development book or a therapy session) into our daily lives, and therefore glean the maximum benefit from it. Perhaps most of all, I recognize that we all, to varying degrees, need impartial guidance in tackling life's travails.

It is because of this that I have evolved a vision of a global wellbeing support system that, above all else, embraces an holistic and personalized approach. I feel that today's world offers so much possibility, but it is also a confusing and lonely place to be sometimes. I believe that we all need support, particularly at a time when real community is dropping away, and we are living in ever less intimate, urban jungles.

This Book

In my view, we are at a 'tipping point', where many people are waking up to the compelling possibility of their lives, and yet simultaneously are recognizing the need for some form of 'support system'. It is to you brave souls, the ones who are no longer interested in following the status quo of a *normal* existence, that I address this book. I invite you to journey with me and discover that it is your birthright to be the master of your own wellbeing.

How do you do this?

My answer in four words is

Wake Up and SOAR

The book is going to express precisely what I mean by this, and then offer some clear, practical guidance about how to integrate the lessons learned into your life. In my view, there are three keys to mastering your wellbeing. The three parts of the book each cover one of the keys:

Part 1: The First Key • Learn To Calm Your Mind • 'Relax'

Part 2: The Second Key • Take Charge of Your Wellbeing • 'Nurture'

Part 3: The Third Key • Pursue Your Dreams • 'Fly'

Each of the three parts of the book also provides a tool for mastering that particular key, and begins with a short story which introduces the tool. Throughout each part of the book I will then refer back to the story (as well as any previous stories), and any key messages, to help you integrate the tool into your daily life.

The three 'tools' are these:

- Wake Up and SOAR

- Your Personal Support System

- The Law Of Magic

Without doubt, the most important message of the book is to learn to calm your mind, using the Wake Up and SOAR tool. This allows you to move from your *normal*, fear-based quality of mind to your *natural*, loving quality of mind. Everything else in the book stems from this.

How To Use The Book

This book is not about theory. I have lived and breathed the experiences that are the basis of all that I have written. I would therefore invite you to see this book as the possibility for your own practical journey. With this in mind, I have a few suggestions with regard to extracting the most from the book:

1   I would encourage you to use a journal. I've used a lot of emboldened and italicized words and phrases within the narrative, which you might want to pay particular attention to, and make notes about.

2   When I read a book, I like to highlight words and phrases, and even though you will be using a journal you might consider doing the same, for emphasis.

3   I would suggest that you journal in the moment that you are thinking or feeling something important, and not wait till you reach the end of a section or chapter. There will be parts of the book which perhaps challenge or inspire you. I would like to encourage you to observe and sense what you are feeling, and then note down what is important for you about the experience.

4   I encourage you to take advantage of the practical sections throughout the book, particularly those accompanying the three tools. I recommend that you respond to these by practicing what is suggested, or responding to questions by writing answers in your journal.

5   I will be constantly referring back to a phrase, or whole section within a previous chapter. I encourage you to do the same, in order to remind yourself of important points, or for the purpose of clarification. To help with this, each chapter has a summary, which offers you an at-a-glance reminder of the main points within the chapter.

6   At the beginning of each of the three parts of the book, I summarize what we have learnt so far, and then briefly outline what is going to be covered in that part of the book.

7   The final chapter, Chapter 9, is an overall summary of the book, and expresses what I feel is most important for you to take away. There is then a What Next? section. This is in respect to what I've said about the 'hot bath' effect. No matter how useful this book is to you (and I truly hope that it is), I would like to take it a stage further, and offer you the possibility for ongoing support.

8   Since your *normal* and *natural* qualities of mind are so fundamental to the essential message, I will continually refer to them throughout the book. My intention is that each time you see these words, you take a moment to reflect on your own 'state of mind'. I shall explain clearly what I mean by this in Part 1 of the book.

It's my observation that people write books such as these for one of two reasons: Firstly, because they are experts in a field, and they want to share their knowledge. Or secondly, because they are passionate about a subject, and recognize that the writing of the book will be an incredible opportunity for their own growth; and it may also, therefore, be of some benefit to others.

I fall into the second category. I am a yogi entrepreneur, who has been inspired to write about how you and I might approach our lives, so that we optimize our possibility for health, happiness and fulfillment. Writing this book has already served me immeasurably. I truly wish that your journey in reading this book be as powerful and transformative for you as it has been for me in researching and writing it.

Notes

1. By Source I am referring to that place within all of us where we meet – beyond race, creed, color, gender – the profound depth of our being.

Part 1

The First Key

Learn To Calm Your Mind

'Relax'

Part 1 of the book is a consideration of the essential problem that we all face as human beings – having a busy mind that frequently leads us on a roller-coaster ride of emotions.

Wake Up and SOAR – the First Tool – allows you to calm your mind at will and therefore relax.

'TAMING THE LAKE MONSTER'

There is an ancient fable about a land beyond time and space. In this forgotten land there was a beautiful lake. All the animals loved to come to her edge and drink from the clear, fresh water, which was said to have special healing powers because her floor was layered with the most beautiful and luminescent crystals.

Deep within the lake everything was serene and perfect, yet the lake was full of sadness. No one had ever seen her true beauty, or the magical crystals in all their glory, since the surface waters of the lake were inhabited by a monster who believed that he was the ruler of this watery kingdom. Whilst he was not dangerous, for he had no teeth or claws, he moved endlessly through the surface waters so that the true beauty of the lake was obscured from view. All day long the monster swam restlessly backwards and forwards across the lake preventing anyone from marvelling at the treasures within. Yet he was not a happy monster, because he was so obsessed with his need to be disruptive.

At night, once there was darkness, the monster slowly sank into sleep and gently came to rest on the floor of the lake where he became one with the serenity all around. Occasionally he stirred during the night and moved around a little, as if swimming in his sleep, so accustomed was he to his daily

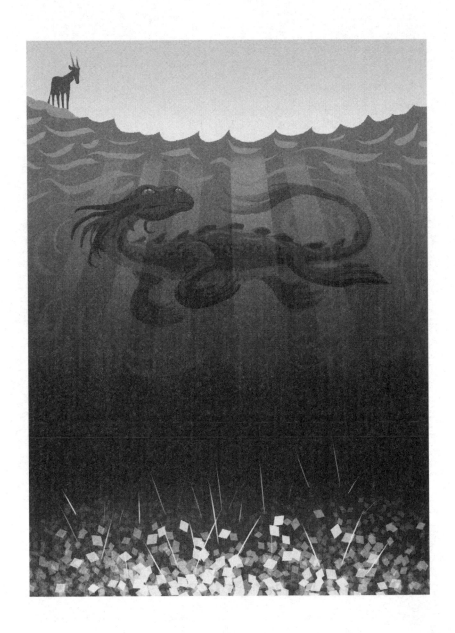

habit of disturbing the calm waters. Unfortunately, though, no one could ever see or appreciate the divine beauty of the lake in the dark of night whilst the monster was sleeping. Even the piercing light of the full moon was not enough to enlighten the depths of the lake.

One day a loud and resonant voice came from the sky and spoke directly to the lake, saying, 'Why are you so sad and why are you not taming this troublesome creature? He is in your waters and it is up to you to train him to be more still. Encourage him to swim more slowly, deep within your waters, so that he does not cause your surface to be so full of waves. Even I, who know of your beauty, am unable to see it with my own eyes, so persistent is this monster in his disruptive ways. Even you cannot know of your own magnificence until you allow it to shine forth for all to see.

With these words the lake felt a deep sense of longing. She decided that she would begin to tame the monster at once, and every day whenever she remembered, she called quietly to him and invited him to swim ever deeper and more slowly, so that her surface waters were less and less disturbed. She showed him that if he behaved more calmly, as he was when restfully asleep, then he too would be happier and more peaceful.

After some time, the monster came to realize that he was not the ruler of the lake, and that he never had been. In fact the monster was very grateful for what he had learned, since he had now found a calmness that was far more pleasant than his restlessly swimming back and forth.

Now, when viewed from the surface, the inner reaches of the lake appeared as a kaleidoscope of color with a myriad of indescribably beautiful reflections. And so it was that the lake awoke and was no longer sad, since she now realized her own beauty. The sky and all of the animals were also able to see her magnificence, and they were especially happy since this reminded them of their own beauty, which they could clearly see reflected in her calm, still waters.

Chapter 1

The Challenge and the Opportunity

Normal vs Natural

In the story overleaf, the monster is a representation of the human mind, and how it tends to seduce us into being lost in thought. He's not a bad monster, just one who is poorly educated. So the message of the story is that we learn to relax through calming our mind.

Because of our own monster's habit of swimming about randomly, it's often the case that we can't see our own inner beauty; and, whether you believe it or not, the beauty is there within us all. The fact that this is sometimes not evident in certain people, is merely a reflection of how busy and distracting their lake monster is.

When the monster is allowed to behave in his normal, bothersome way, we are not very happy. Research undertaken at Harvard University in 2010, revealed that

> *'People spend 46.9 percent of their waking hours thinking about something other than what they're doing, and this mind-wandering typically makes them unhappy.'*[1]

Since happiness and health go hand in hand, when we're not very happy, we tend not to be very healthy either. So the biggest problem that we face in life today is not global warming, our challenging relationships with others, or having less money than we would ideally like to have, but rather that our mind is racing out of control. Some of us already know this, but either we've never considered that we can do anything about it, or if we have, we don't know where to begin.

I would like to suggest, however, that this is a huge and magnificent opportunity, since if we can tame our own lake monster, and we can, then we become the masters of our own health and happiness.

I invite you to consider this for a moment.

However, the rub is this – taming the lake monster is a tricky affair. We are so conditioned in the way that we think, speak and act that in some ways we behave more like robots than sentient beings at the top of the food chain. For much of the time, we give most of our attention to the monster, allowing it to disturb the calm waters of our being. This is, for many of us, what we might call the *normal* state.

Yet this is not our *natural* human state.

Our *natural* state is to be vibrantly alive, neither stressed nor causing stress to others. Ancient tribes, at least the smarter ones, existed in small enclaves where sustainability and community were part of the fabric of their existence. They flourished, and yet lived utterly in harmony with nature. They took just enough for their needs, and willingly gave back, or shared, what they didn't need. They were living naturally.

Think of it like the breath. We need to inhale to feed our body with what it needs, thereby taking care of ourselves, so that we can then exhale what we don't need, thereby giving back to life. It is our *natural* human state to breathe. It is also *natural* to take good care of ourselves and therefore want to give of ourselves to others. But due to life's circumstances, many of us have, to a greater or lesser extent, been programed into the *normal* state, where we tend to be contracted and less compassionate towards ourselves and others.

Our *natural* state is where, through calmness of mind, we breathe efficiently, take care of the needs of our body and avoid stress. In the *normal* state we're frequently lost in thought, and therefore breathe less fully than we need to, are perhaps careless with the needs of our body, and experience stress.

We humans were born with certain capabilities that are unique to us. We have great intelligence, and are self-reflective, meaning that we can observe and analyze our own behavior and then come to certain informed conclusions.

We are capable of realizing when we are in the *normal* state, and we have the power to transcend this and return to our *natural* state. It's *normal* that our lake monster is thrashing about, bit it's *natural* that we learn to calm him and remember our inner peace of being.

The Predominant Trends of Today

We are in the midst of the most profound financial, social and political shift in modern history – every area of human life is in an accelerated state of flux, and the terrain is changing fast. It is clear that the stressors affecting human beings in this 21st century are growing in force and number. Yet so too are the possibilities for countering these issues.

There are distinct, even polarized, trends which are emerging in today's world: the *normal* 'problem trends', and the *natural* 'solution trends'.

The Normal *'Problem Trends'*

1. *Communality and real intimacy are rapidly dwindling for many people*
Since the Industrial Revolution, and now in the midst of the Digital Age, communality and intimacy are rapidly diminishing for many of us. We have forgotten what it is like to live in small manageable clusters of

people, which nurture a healthy sense of 'belonging to the tribe'. We are so busy rushing everywhere, at the beck and call of our mobile devices.

The modern 'urban grind' is no longer a pejorative description, but more an accepted trade-off between our 'desire for more', and a sacrifice of our health and wellbeing, and therefore also our *natural* state. With this, there is a growing tendency for greed and selfishness, since we are very focused on what will make *me* feel good. Perhaps inevitably as people increasingly live in vast urban clusters, and the Digital Age burgeons, there is a sense that 'Me' is prevailing over 'We'.

2. We are increasingly divorced from Mother Nature

The distractions of the Digital Age mean that we are ever more divorced from Mother Nature. Most of us live in urban jungles characterized by ever-greater demands and expectations, where communication is measured in milliseconds and life pressures are high. Many of us living in the modern world today have a number of digital devices which render us 'on call' 24/7, and we are therefore rarely in 'off' mode.

In other words, our 'lake monster' is stimulated and encouraged to be active, and we endlessly fall back into a *normal* quality of mind.

It's very hard to resist the temptation to react to texts, messages and emails the minute that we are alerted to their arrival. This may well reveal a deeper desire – that of feeling wanted or important. Perhaps because of this, as well as our tendency towards habitual behavioral patterns, we often react to digital beeps and pings without really considering whether we need to respond immediately or not.

3. We have a growing tendency to delegate responsibility to others

Self-responsibility has been eschewed in favor of endlessly consulting experts, and many people are losing their intuitive sense of how to take care of themselves. There is a corresponding global trend of governments and the 'powers that be' exerting ever more control. Civil liberties are being eroded on the pretext of countering terrorism and civil disobedience.

Having lost touch with Mother Nature, we have also lost touch with our own inner nature, and sense of intuition. We easily fall into a sheep-like mentality, where the status quo perspective on life makes our behavior predictable and manageable.

4. The quality of our food and drink is increasingly compromised

The goodness of what we eat and drink is diminishing. Foodstuffs which are highly processed, and full of artificial sweeteners, colorants and additives, are simply not conducive to a healthy gut or immune system.

A growing number of herbicides, pesticides, preservatives, and many other unspecified chemicals and pollutants are entering the earth's soil, water, and air. This issue is compounded by GM farming and other such practices, purportedly intended to solve the food supply problem.

5. Economic troubles, poverty and inequality abound

Economic growth in the so-called developed world is likely to be severely limited (at least for the next few years), and businesses, organizations and individuals need to be circumspect about the future.

Many humans are desperately poor, either herded together in urban slums or remote rural dwellings. These people lack education and the basic means to take care of themselves and their families with any dignity.

- The United Nations Food and Agriculture Organization estimates that about 805 million, or 11 per cent of the world's population, were suffering from chronic undernourishment in 2012–14
- 791 million of these lived in developing world countries
- Under-nutrition was the cause of 3.1 million child deaths annually, or 45 per cent of all child deaths in 2011[2]

Whilst poverty and lack of basic amenities for a 'decent' life are, in percentage terms, predominantly the curse of developing nations, the developed world also has major problems relating to poverty and health:

- 3.7 million children were living in poverty in the UK in 2013–14. i.e. 28 per cent of children[3]
- 4 out of 5 US adults struggle with joblessness, near-poverty or reliance on welfare for at least parts of their lives[4]

In spite of the progress made in many regions of the world, sexism, racism and fundamentalism are still major global issues; there is, perhaps, no better example than this, of a mind, or minds, which are so fully under the spell of their conditioned, *normal* state of mind.

6. We are having an increasingly negative impact upon our earthly biosphere

This is reaching a state of emergency today. Over the last 100 years or so, there has been a waning of biodiversity, with many species of plants and animals endangered or extinct, and this trend is accelerating fast. There is also a seemingly intractable problem of pollution by industry and individuals alike, with CO_2 emissions rising off the scale. Whether we humans are the key to this issue or not, we are, at the very least, feeding the problem. Our rivers, lakes and seas are increasingly polluted, and we have no effective way of dealing with the mountains of waste that we are producing.

That we are still reliant upon fossil fuels in this age of scientific supremacy is embarrassing. Sustainability is losing the battle against greed and excessive consumption.

7. We are experiencing a global epidemic of stress and chronic disease

Due to the previous six trends, we are experiencing a profound knock-on effect – stress, addiction, anxiety and depression are all on the increase. According to the American Institute of Stress, stress is the basic cause of 60 per cent of all human illness and disease. Apart from acute conditions there are a myriad of other unpleasant and debilitating conditions which result from stress, such as colds and flu, asthma, stomach ulcers, kidney stones, post-traumatic stress disorder, irritable bowel syndrome, depression, eczema and other skin disorders.

Addiction is so common-place today as to be the norm rather than the exception. Almost everyone is addicted to something – sugar, food, alcohol, cigarettes, drugs, sex, mobile phones, computers, money and so on. Most of us have some form of 'crutch' that we rely on as a part of our daily routine in order to be distracted, to unwind or to help us deal with difficult times.

The likelihood is that many people are going to feel increasingly less healthy in the coming years, since, like the Earth's biosphere, our bodily systems are suffering from toxic overload – mentally, emotionally and physically. Unfortunately, healthcare services and the western clinical model of medicine which exists today are woefully inadequate to deal with the challenge of chronic disease and stress. On top of this, the worldwide issue of funding public healthcare is at crisis point, even in countries which have traditionally prided themselves in having excellent welfare services.

- 3 out of 4 doctor's visits in the US are for stress-related ailments (American Institute Of Stress)
- The proportion of deaths due to non-communicable disease is projected to rise from 59 per cent in 2002 to 69 per cent in 2030[5]
- Between 1983 and 2008, diabetes increased seven-fold, from 35m to 240m people[6]

- In 2012 in the US, about 50 per cent of all adults (117m) had one or more chronic health conditions, and 25 per cent of adults had two or more; in 2010 70 per cent of deaths were due to chronic diseases – two of these, heart disease and cancer, accounted for nearly 48 per cent of all deaths[7]
- According to the World Health Organization, in 2015 there were about 2.3 billion overweight people aged 15 and above, and over 700 million obese people worldwide[8]

The Natural *'Solution Trends'*

1. The incredible opportunity offered by the Digital Age

The Digital Age has provided us with powerful tools for communicating all that is good and beautiful about life. Indeed, it allows us to muster ourselves into tribes which bring about positive transformation – for example, Avaaz (an advocacy group comprising an on-line community of over 25 million people), Greenpeace and many other eco-movements the world over.

Researching and writing this book would have been much harder without the benefit of the internet. Tools such as Google, YouTube, Wikipedia, Facebook, Twitter, Instagram and many other social networking sites bring mountains of information to the fore. Important and sensitive issues are much less likely to be brushed under the carpet, and the average person is generally far more informed than ever before.

When we are in our *natural* state of mind, our smart phones and ubiquitous connectivity with the WWW are incredibly potent tools. From this perspective, the Digital Age facilitates all the other trends which follow, since it provides both the information required as well as the means for their emergence and flowering.

2. Many people are awakening to the need for a shift from 'Me' to 'We'

There is a growing realization that co-operation, not competition, is the way forward. This is being triggered by various factors, not least of which is the suffering and inequality that it so palpable across the globe today.

The Digital Age, and particularly social media, has caused millions of people to wake up to the need to care for the billions of people who are poor, uneducated and helpless in the world. This won't resolve all issues around poverty and inequality, but it is having a vital impact.

Sexism, racism and fundamentalism will never entirely disappear, in my view, but once again the advent of the internet means that important and sensitive issues can no longer be ignored. We are all so much more aware of the injustices of the world, and there are so many charities, advocacy groups, NGOs and philanthropic organizations devoted to addressing matters of human inequality.

This trend is greatly supported by the way in which modern science is validating ancient wisdom, recognizing and 'proving' so much of that which has been intuited and taught in the great healing arts for millennia. Ancient wisdom is grounded in Mother Nature, teaching that we are 'all one', and that everything in life therefore affects everything else.

3. There is a growing trend towards self-responsibility
Across the globe, many of us are increasingly choosing to be less dependent upon others for our wellbeing. We realize that governments and all other organizations which we perhaps previously saw as the ultimate authority, are as fraught with human fallibility as each one of us. This gives us a whole new sense of responsibility for ourselves.

There is a growing trend of people choosing to live in smaller communities amidst nature. I myself choose to live in quiet, out-of-the-way places, which are far more harmonious and community-minded than the urban alternative. Amongst such communities, there is recognition of our essential unity, and ideas of difference based on race, creed, color and so on are far less evident.

Greed and selfishness don't disappear, for sure, but in my experience our awareness of them is heightened. We are much clearer about our role in the bigger picture of life when we live in small communities.

4. We are seeing the emergence of a new perspective on health and wellbeing
In much the same way that the 'problem trends' have created the explosion in stress and chronic disease globally, the preceding three 'solution trends' are causing an awakening to the fact that

We are the masters of our health and happiness

The holistic wellbeing industry burgeons, and many humans are waking up to the realization that not only can they be in charge of their own wellbeing and sense of aliveness, but also that disease prevention is a better course of action than cure.

We seem to be realizing that something must give in this 'game of life', and more and more people are seeking soul sanctuaries in the form of yoga classes and retreats, detox courses and retreats, and healthy living options.

The Yoga Phenomenon
Since it has no one founder, ultimate authority or racial bias, yoga 'talks' to a vast, and varied, audience of hundreds of millions of people, and inspires them to be more self-reliant. For most people, yoga is a group class which leaves you feeling deeply relaxed. Those who become committed often develop their own personal practice and explore the full benefits of yoga, which cover the whole of the human lifestyle. Increasing numbers of students are now also becoming teachers – the benefits of which are not just a new career path, but also a deepening of one's own practice.

Yoga therapy, or 'yoga as medicine', is forecast to be one of the major wellbeing trends of the coming years. According to a 2008 study by 'Research and Markets'

- 6 per cent or nearly 14 million Americans say that a doctor or therapist has recommended yoga to them
- 45 per cent of all adult Americans agree that yoga would be beneficial if they were undergoing treatment for a medical condition

---

Usually practiced one to one, this is the logical outcome of applying yogic principles to chronic problems, sickness prevention and the attainment of optimal health and happiness. The possibility for diagnosing imbalances within clients and prescribing yogic practices and lifestyle guidelines, is providing a potent form of complementary medicine. In recognition of this, Kaitlin Quistgaard, editor in chief of *Yoga Journal*, (the most distributed yoga magazine today) said:

> *'Yoga as medicine represents the next great yoga wave. In the next few years, we will be seeing a lot more yoga in healthcare settings and more yoga recommended by the medical community, as new research shows that yoga is a valuable therapeutic tool for many health conditions.'[9]*

Detox and Rejuvenation
These are words which are fast catching the imagination of the urban populous, and people are ever more aware of the need to counteract the harmful toxic overload of today's lifestyles. Matthias Dehne, of 'The Healthy Healing Clinic Goa' has this to say on the matter:

> *'Worldwide, detoxification programs and protocols are the trend in preventive medicine. Detox is in demand. Why? Simple, because it addresses a need. More and more people are becoming aware that we live in a toxic world.'*

Nutrition and Diet
Not surprisingly, nutrition has become a point of discussion throughout all strata of society, and whilst there is often a lack of consensus, the

all-important conversations are going on, and are now too deeply established to merely evaporate.

Many people are now aware of the problems of industrialized food and GMO, and are opting for free-range or pasture-fed, organic and natural alternatives.

Complementary and Alternative Therapies, and Integrative Medicine
We are in the age of complementary and alternative medicine and therapies. Many people are now opting for preventative measures, holistic alternatives to traditional, medical practices and a more integrative approach to medicine.

Integrative medicine (the marriage of traditional, western medical practices with holistic healing systems) offers a powerful way of embracing the body's natural healing capacity, whilst recognizing that we are all unique. There are clinics and medical centers adopting this approach throughout the world today. I believe that this is a key element of future medicine.

What Can We Learn From Today's Predominant Trends?

A Call For Action

In spite of the potency of the *natural* solution trends, the *normal* problem trends are having a disastrous impact on the health and happiness of many human beings, not to mention the abuse of our biosphere.

In my view, many of the problems within human society today are rooted in the first two of **The *Normal* 'Problem Trends'**:

1 *'Communality and real intimacy are rapidly dwindling for many people'*

2 *'We are increasingly divorced from Mother Nature'*

We live in an age of loneliness, where we've forgotten our essential need to belong to a tribe. We are also neglecting Mother Nature, and therefore our own inner nature; because of this, we are increasingly greedy and consuming like crazy.

Planet Earth is under no threat, of course, because Mother Nature merely needs to sneeze and we will all be blown into oblivion. She is not deeply affected by our ignorant actions.

No, the problem is not our planet, it is we, the human race, who are in peril. If we fail to alter our current trajectory, based on a *normal* mindset of greed, scarcity and intolerance, then we will find ourselves on a planet that is ever less habitable.

The Evolutionary Necessity

We are witnessing a time of incredible transformation. In many ways, we are privileged to live at this time. History is unfolding at breakneck speed before our eyes, and we are being presented with a choice:

Are we ready to take charge of our health and happiness, realizing that we have a lake monster, and that we can choose to calm him? Are we ready to 'Wake Up and SOAR'?

Or will we continue to drift along the pathways of our lives, hoping that something or someone is going to make everything ok by pressing a magical 'reset' button?

We are all being urged to adopt a radical new perspective about life and our part in it. In modern marketing parlance we might call this a 'tipping point'.

In his acclaimed book *The Tipping Point*, Malcolm Gladwell eloquently expresses what a tipping point is: 'The tipping point is the moment of critical mass, the threshold, the boiling point.' He likens the tipping point to the spread of an epidemic. He also highlights the three characteristics, or rules, of the phenomenon – 'The law of the few, the stickiness factor and the power of context.'

In my words, the three factors, or rules, are

- A small number of influential people can be agents of profound change
- The message or mission must be simple and memorable
- Timing and circumstances must be opportune

So this tells us clearly what to look out for in identifying a potential tipping point.

If you take a good, honest look at the world today, perhaps you see the same as I do, that many of us are woefully ignorant about sustainability. Unfortunately, this means that big businesses and governments, who after all are made up of individuals like you and me, are taking our beautiful planet for granted. My feeling is that the root cause of this is our predilection for falling into a *normal*, fearful state of being, rather than a *natural*, loving one.

I'm a huge fan of the Digital Age, and yet I see it as a double-edged sword, since it both offers great opportunity, and yet also increases our tendency towards stress and disease. This latter tendency is both direct, in that we can easily become further conditioned into *normal*, fearful thinking, and also indirect, in the sense that having our faces stuck in some form of 'smart device' all day long, is probably not so good for us.

Yet, if we observe the *normal* 'problem' trends closely, don't we have the ingredients for a tipping point? In fact, can we perhaps see that the 'tip' is well under way, in the form of the *natural* 'solution trends'?

If we use the above characteristics of a tipping point:

The small number of influential people is in fact millions of concerned people (YOU), armed with supremely powerful mobile devices and apps, and the internet.

The message, or mission, which must be simple and memorable is circling the globe in the digital ether, and is as potent as any virus and very much simpler to understand:

> *'We are supremely potent beings with the capacity to be the masters of our own wellbeing. Many of us are increasingly seeking self-responsibility, and the opportunity to nudge human evolution in a positive direction by rising to the challenge of being the best that we can be.'*

The timing and circumstances – The trajectory of humankind is not a positive one, with stress and chronic disease spiraling out of control, widespread inequality, civil unrest and war, and a biosphere which is seriously compromised.

So whilst the *normal*, problem trends might at first paint a bleak picture, I see them as triggers (the evolutionary necessity) for the raising of human consciousness (the *natural*, solution trends).

Who would have dreamt ten years ago that acupuncture would be offered on the UK National Health Service today? And who could have predicted that the new Prime Minister of India, Narendra Modi, would be so brilliantly selling yoga to the world, including the creation of an 'International Day of Yoga'?

I believe, as do many, that we have the possibility to take a profound step forward in human evolution. These kinds of extremes of ignorance and suffering (the *normal* 'problem' trends) have previously caused seminal shifts in human history, because they ignite the human imagination and encourage self-responsibility. The 'Great Depression' of the 1930s, and the two World Wars in the last century, were good examples of this, where countries united in a common cause.

Today, a new collective consciousness is emerging, precisely because so many of us are concerned about the trajectory of the human race. I feel that we're being pushed to question our individual and collective purposes more than ever before, and to realize that the problems we're facing actually represent a magnificent opportunity:

The Problem (Normal *State*)

We frequently seem to be in resistance to nature's flow; many of us don't appear to be functioning as though we are part of the same human tribe. We increasingly seek to push the limits of this beautiful symphony called life, grabbing greedily at Mother Nature's resources; polluting the air and water one moment, then consuming it the next; and coveting all that we have not yet branded as ours.

The Opportunity (Natural *State*)

We have the possibility to Wake Up. Only we, the human race, can judiciously reflect upon our actions and those of others, override our normal, primal instincts and inclinations, and consciously decide upon a wiser course of action. We are the masters of our own wellbeing, and once we feel well, we can love all others like brothers and sisters, and take good care of our beautiful planet. In other words, we are able to flow with life just like the rest of nature.

It seems sad that we humans need to reach the point of almost destroying our biosphere, before we wake up to our magical possibility here on Earth. Yet this is the way of Mother Nature – an endless cycle of cause and effect. Our current plight is the evolutionary necessity for us to rise to the magnificent challenge that stands before us. I believe passionately that we are capable of so much more than we imagine. It is with this passion and heartfelt belief that I invite you to journey with me, and discover the compelling possibility of your life.

What I feel is vital to understand is that the solution to humankind's 'problem', begins within each one of us. Hence, as Satyananda says, we must take care of 'inner ecology before outer ecology'.

Quality of Mind

If a group of us view the same image or event, we will all perceive things slightly differently. The differences may be subtle, but they will be there nonetheless. Each of our minds is capable of vastly differing perspectives. What we're 'seeing' is subject to what I'm going to call our individual quality (or state) of mind.

If you take a moment to consider it, you'll realize that the quality of your mind plays a role in everything that you think, feel, say and do. In fact, it underlies the totality of your life experience, and is therefore at the epicenter of your health and happiness.

Why do I say this?

Our mind is like the software which runs the hardware of our brain; and quality of mind is just another way of saying our degree of consciousness. By which I mean the extent to which we are here in this present moment and choosing where we put our attention. So the *normal* and *natural* states are qualities of mind, which describe our level of consciousness.

It is *natural* for us to have a quality of mind characterized by ease and flow, with a lack of resistance to what is arising. Yet, it's also normal for unconsciousness[10] to creep up on us. In my experience, the *normal* state of mind resides as a subtle haze that limits my creativity and imagination; but it can also grow to become a dense fog which totally shrouds my capacity for clear thinking.

The way I see it, is that in our *natural* state we will be treating our bodies and minds as the temples that they are, and considerably increasing the possibility for a happy and healthy life. Unfortunately, though, most of us spend much of our time in a more *normal*, unconscious state of mind, and therefore fail to intuit our needs in order to attain, or maintain, optimal wellbeing.

So, the *natural* state is an awakened quality of mind offering unlimited possibility; whereas the *normal* state is that same magnificent possibility 'contracted'. Using the example of the story, our *natural* quality of mind is the beautiful, expansive lake, which when disrupted by the lake monster becomes murky and unclear, defaulting to its *normal* state.

So how is our quality of mind determined?

Ultimately this is a mystery, and therefore I am not really able to explain it. What I can say, though, is that our quality of mind seems to have been influenced by the way in which we've internalized all that's happened to us throughout our lives – our past conditioning. This past conditioning has programed our 'software' (mind), to produce innumerable habits, many of which don't serve us. The programing began way back when we were babies in our cots and push chairs, as we were being taught how to 'see the world' by our parents and siblings.

> If you think about some of your daily activities (those things which might feel repetitive, boring or tiresome), such as brushing your teeth, traveling to work, or putting out the rubbish, can you sense that you are frequently running on autopilot?

These moments when we've 'zoned-out', or are lost in conditioned thought, are what I mean by a *normal* state of mind. I think that for many of us, this has become our default setting. I'm not suggesting that we're cursed with being stuck in a *normal* state of mind, but that we have the tendency to be somewhat contracted more often than not. This creates a number of recognizable human tendencies:

Delegation of Responsibility

Many of us have clearly lost the intuitive discernment that allows us to determine the best course of action when faced with life's everyday challenges. Hence, when we are sick, we generally turn to medical experts to cure us, without giving thought to our part in the healing process.

This *normal* quality of mind is beautifully expressed in the Hollywood film, *The Matrix*, when the character Morpheus says to Neo:

> '*You have to understand, most of these people are not ready to be unplugged ... and many of them are so injured, so hopelessly dependent on the system, that they will fight to protect it.*'

Fearful vs Loving

In the Native American culture of the Cherokee tribe, *normal* and *natural* were likened to two wolves within us:

> '*There is a battle of two wolves inside us all. One is evil. It is anger, jealousy, greed, resentment, lies, inferiority and ego. The other is good. It is joy, peace, love, hope, humility, kindness, empathy and truth.*
> *The wolf that wins? The one you feed.*'

John Lennon said the same thing with different words, where he spoke of fear and love, rather than good and evil:

> '*There are two basic motivating forces: fear and love. When we are afraid, we pull back from life. When we are in love, we open to all that life has to offer with passion, excitement, and acceptance ...*'

Isn't this also what the Bible means by heaven and hell – our capacity for experiencing life as peaceful and joyful, or as disturbing and painful?

'Story': The Inner Dialogue of Your Mind

Just take a moment now to breathe slowly and consciously, and observe what is happening within your being.

Can you notice the arising of thoughts?

These might appear as a stream of words like an inner dialogue, or perhaps as moving images. If you watch for a while, you may notice that if left unattended, these thoughts are often random.

Now imagine a swimming-pool cleaning machine that is unmanned and flailing around in the water, randomly sucking up bits of leaves and debris from the pool's bottom. These leaves and debris then pass through the pool's filtration system, and 'color' it.

In the same way, when you're in a *normal* state of mind, your attention often meanders randomly through the databank of your memories, picking up bits here and there. Whichever thoughts catch your attention most, 'color' the filter through which your mind then operates. These thoughts are then reflected in your body as emotions. If you merely notice these thoughts and emotions, then all is well. But if you are attracted, and therefore somehow attached to them, then you make them into a story, one which endlessly grabs at your attention. It's the extent to which you live in these stories that determines your quality of mind, and therefore also your quality of life.

Maybe you can even sense right now that your mind is talking to you, telling you that you agree or disagree with what I'm saying?

Suffering

Due to the habit which most of us have, of projecting our story onto the screen of life, what happens around us may sometimes feel 'wrong' or 'uncomfortable', since we are not seeing or accepting the reality of a situation. A *normal* quality of mind, therefore, tends to create inner resistance, however subtle, and thus also degrees of suffering.

> **Suffering arises from our unwillingness to see,**
> **and accept, life as it actually is**

Can you think of a recent situation where you've suffered?

Can you see that the suffering was due to you not accepting something?

Shakespeare famously said, 'The problem is the others!' In other words, what other people say and do, and what arises around us, will often not match with our pre-conceived ideas (our story) of how things 'should be', based on our inner beliefs.

Hence the religious, political and social discord that we see playing itself out around the globe. Righteousness, arrogance and ignorance will quickly descend into racism, hatred and fundamentalism, if left unchecked.

Desires and Addictions

Because of our unique conditioning, our various stories generate endless desires – desire for more money, a different partner, to look slimmer and so on. My observation is that we generally desire whatever it is that we think will make us happy. As I said in the *Normal* 'Problem Trends' section:

> *'Addiction is so common-place today, as to be the norm rather than the exception. Almost everyone is addicted to something – sugar, food, alcohol, cigarettes, drugs, sex, mobile phones, computers, money and so on. Most of us have some form of "crutch" that we rely on as a part of our daily routine in order to be distracted, to unwind, or to help us to deal with difficult times.'*

What the wise sages of old tell us on this subject is that the reason we so obsessively pursue our superficial desires is that, once fulfilled, they bring a temporary respite from our noisy mind. Beneath our superficial desires is the fundamental longing for the mind to be quiet and in peace – our *natural* state.

I don't think that many of us question ourselves very deeply, and we continue to be seduced by the superficial 'blip' of calm and happiness that results from our habitual pursuit of worldly pleasures. Through unconsciousness we habitually attach to our stories, following the twists and turns of our compelling desires from one minute to the next.

Please don't just believe what I'm saying though. Instead, I invite you to test this for yourself and see if it's true. I'm saying it because I have tested it, and this is how it is for me.

Stress

When we're absorbed in our inner story (*normal* state), we're not choosing where to put our attention. Being lost in unsolicited thought is like resisting this present moment. In this state, our life force doesn't flow freely. The more absorbing and emotion-inducing our story, the more our breath will be contracted, and the greater the tension, or stress, that we will experience. If this stress persists, it becomes increasingly depleting.

**When we resist this present moment by attaching to a story,
we create inner tension, or stress**

Applying too much stress to anything will weaken it. If you take a spoon, and repeatedly bend it one way and then the other, you 'stress' it, and eventually it will snap. If you observe human beings, you'll see that it works the same way with us.

'Fight or flight'

When we were 'hunter-gatherers' and we faced fierce animals, there was a vital animal instinct at play, that of survival – escape or be killed!

Like all other animals, we humans are equipped with a brilliant survival mechanism called 'fight or flight' – in anatomy and physiology this is termed the sympathetic nervous system. This emergency mechanism allows us to deal with life-threatening situations quite brilliantly, by allowing us to mobilize a huge amount of energy rapidly.

We are equipped to either 'fight the beast', or to high-tail it away with great speed. When our brain senses danger it instantaneously releases a cocktail of chemicals such as adrenalin and cortisol into the blood stream, causing a dramatic physiological response:

> Blood pressure rises, muscles tense, breathing becomes shallow and rapid, digestion stops, pupils dilate, awareness intensifies, sight sharpens, impulses quicken, perception of pain diminishes, and our immune system is mobilized. All systems go on full alert, and we become prepared physically and mentally for fight or flight, as we scan our surroundings for the 'enemy'.

This is diametrically opposed to the normal functioning of our bodily rhythm, where 90 per cent of our energy is devoted to growth and renewal – the maintenance of homeostasis. Fight or flight is a program which shuts down these vital functions as it is geared exclusively towards dealing with the perceived danger.

Below is a quote from an article by Neil F. Neimark, MD, of the Mind/Body Education Center, which expresses the negative and limiting implications when our survival mechanism is inappropriately triggered:

'When our fight or flight system is activated, we tend to perceive everything in our environment as a possible threat to our survival. By its very nature, the fight or flight system bypasses our rational mind, where our more well thought-out beliefs exist, and moves us into "attack" mode.'[11]

When you are in this state, your 'filter' is clouded by fearful thoughts of what might go wrong, or what you yourself are perhaps doing wrong. Like airport security during a terrorist threat, you are on the lookout for possible danger.

When the lens through which you see the world is so narrow and contracted, you are really only focused on survival. Your heart is not open, and you are not thinking clearly. Your ability to feel compassion or to have loving thoughts towards others is minimized. There is really no possibility for cultivating inner, or outer, harmony when you are locked into survival mode.

There are actually two components to the survival mechanism – the sympathetic nervous system and the parasympathetic nervous system. The sympathetic nervous system functions like the accelerator pedal in a car. It triggers the fight-or-flight response, providing the body with a burst of energy so that it can respond to perceived dangers, or the need for rapid action. The parasympathetic nervous system acts like a brake, and promotes the 'rest-and-digest' response that calms the body down after the danger has passed.

In ancient times man came face to face with grizzly bears and saber-toothed tigers as part of his normal hunter-gatherer routine. Yet once the danger had passed, his auto-response mechanism would switch off and his bodily rhythms would return to normal thanks to his parasympathetic nervous system.

If you observe animals, you'll see these two aspects of the survival mechanism at play. You don't even need to be in the wild to observe this.

You can see it with ducks in a pond, or even with domesticated cats and dogs. Intermittently they will challenge one another, and even fight quite aggressively. But once the fight is over, all those involved will flap their wings, or shake their torsos vigorously, to release the excess energy which results from the injection of adrenalin and cortisol into their systems.

In the case of human mental and emotional stress, precisely the same physical cues are delivered, and so – blood pressure rises, muscles tense, breathing becomes shallow and rapid, digestion stops, the immune system is mobilized, and all systems go on full alert. Once the trigger is no longer active, and our parasympathetic nervous system takes over, we calm down. But if the stress is persistent, or regular, then the correct functioning of all of the bodily systems is compromised.

I can't help but notice how well 'fight or flight' describes the greatest affliction of our modern-day society, wherein our bodies are endlessly confused into believing that there is a threat. This places enormous stress on all levels of our being – mental, physical and emotional. If this stress remains unchecked, then chronic physical illness and premature aging will result. This, in my view, reveals the best non-surgical aid to diminishing the aging process – de-stress :)

You will probably notice how perfectly the two components of the survival mechanism – the sympathetic nervous system (accelerator) and the parasympathetic nervous system (brake) – seem to correspond with *normal* and *natural*. It is normal that we tense up and go on full alert when a wild animal is standing in front of us, but it is *natural* that we return to a calm, restful state, as soon as the danger has passed.

The *normal* state renders us contracted, akin to survival mode, whereas our *natural* state is an expansive one that allows us to relax and feel good. The problem is that when we are not taking responsibility for observing our quality of mind, we frequently fall to a default setting of *normal*.

Whilst calling the mind a 'monster' in my story 'Taming the Lake Monster' might seem a little harsh, it is really an acknowledgment of the fact that dealing with our mind is sometimes not unlike confronting a wild beast, albeit one without claws and teeth :).

The Modern-Day Plague

I believe that for many people today, the *normal*, fear-based state of mind is predominant, and therefore also a semi-permanent state of fight or flight. The lake monster is thrashing about, and we are giving him all of our attention.

Modern urban living causes us to be bombarded with mental, physical and emotional tension – our food is industrialized and 'denatured', our water and air are full of toxins, and we live in a digital age where time is measured in milliseconds and we feel the pressure to do more, more quickly. You can perhaps imagine how depleting and stressful this is for our body-mind.[12] It's not surprising, therefore, that chronic disease and stress are spiraling out of control.

Stress, in its multifarious forms, is a part of nature. Its origins may be traced way back to our early evolution, as we have just seen with 'fight or flight'. However, aside from times of great natural disaster, it would

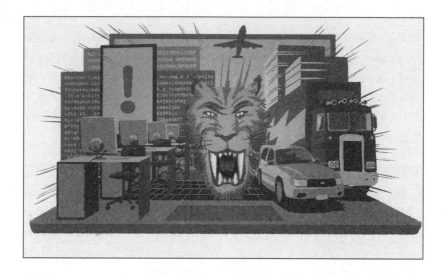

seem as though stress has never figured quite so prominently as it does in today's epidemic proportions.

When stressed, we are more likely to be reactive, perhaps making us more selfish, greedy, or lacking in compassion for our fellow brothers and sisters. We are also more likely to make poor lifestyle choices that do not support us, wherein further stress and perhaps disease are the inevitable consequence.

Because we have seen the gruesome pictures of blackened lungs, and are endlessly confronted with 'warnings of death' on cigarette packets, we are all very much aware of the dangers of smoking. However, the things which trigger our stress mechanism today are experienced so regularly as to dull our awareness of their existence and potential harm.

Whilst ancient man certainly faced huge threats to his survival on a near daily basis, our 21st-century lifestyles have heralded a modern-day plague which is equally threatening, but behaves like a silent stalker. Surprising though it may seem, when a frog is in water that is slowly boiled, it doesn't jump out to save itself. Just as the boiling water will slowly kill the frog, so our modern lifestyles may well be slowly killing us.

The triggers for our stress are so common place, as to cause prevailing stress levels unlike anything seen before in recorded human history. If we exclude the ravages of war, up to 200 years ago, old age was a common cause of death – hence the coroner's report might well have read, 'died of natural causes'. Today, that option is not often open to the coroner, since we almost all die of cancer, heart disease and stroke.

Yes, we generally live for longer these days (though this trend is potentially going to reverse due to global trends of obesity and chronic disease) because of improved standards of sanitation, and drugs designed to 'keep us alive'. But the fact remains that we die 'diseased' due to the myriad of stressors that have wrought havoc upon our wellbeing for a sustained period of time.

So why have so many people become so stressed in this modern era?

There are perhaps two reasons for this:

1. The stressors that we confront have evolved

Whilst our survival mechanism has probably remained unaltered for millennia – after all, it works extremely well regarding the task for which it was created – the nature and extent of the stressors that we confront have evolved markedly.

In the last few decades, particularly, we have seen the complexity of life and the myriad forms of information input multiply dramatically. If you consider many of the influential structures within society today, such as politics, business, religion or the media, and ask yourself the question:

> *'Are these organizations essentially emanating a calm, loving and relaxed vibration; or are their actions generally eliciting fear, anxiety, confusion and doubt?'*

Perhaps you sense the general trend towards the latter. Many of us feel a pressure to be a certain way – 'do more, be more, have more, improve, get slimmer, be more attractive, try harder', and so on. It would seem that we are more manageable within the prevailing systems, when our quality of mind tends towards fear and uncertainty. In this state, we are consuming like crazy, and delegating our responsibility to those we believe know better than we do.

For example, many pregnant women today have lost their sense of how best to nurture their own babies, instead they read books, attend courses, and worry about whether they are 'doing it right'.

2. The complexity of our minds has evolved

The complexity of our minds and their corresponding ability to imagine and fully enact the drama of endless mind-made stories has also evolved immensely. Our advanced mind's capacity for complex and analytical thought creates giga-bytes of mental pictures (memories) that 'appear real' to the brain, and which frequently trigger our primitive survival response.

If there is someone in your life who is verbally abusive to you, then every time that you interact with them, or perhaps even just think about them, you are likely to have powerful, negative memories running through your thoughts. Your brain interprets these thoughts as a threat, since it cannot differentiate between a 'real threat' – a grizzly bear in your pathway, and an 'imagined threat' – someone who you are imagining to be shouting aggressively at you. Through endless scenarios such as this, your body's survival mode may well be triggered on a regular basis.

Our modern minds, so well fed with fearful or anxious thoughts, cause our systems to believe that they need to regularly go into 'survival' mode, and this is far more pernicious than a plague, or even war, since the effects are mostly hidden. It is like the invisible enemy, until that is, the effects have compounded sufficiently to produce physical symptoms.

- When you take a short break from city living, do you notice how wound up you have become?
- Are you aware of the stressors around you?
- Can you sense that advertising and societal pressure sometimes make you feel fearful, disempowered, inadequate or ignorant?
- Do you sometimes feel overwhelmed by the complexity of your life?
- Do you yearn for a simpler way of life?

Stress and Chronic Disease

In the modern era, our normal habits tend to cause high levels of imbalance, leading to stress. The degree of stress is often such that our natural cleansing and renewal mechanisms require support. Most of us realize that stress is unhealthy, a fact borne out by voluminous amounts of current research demonstrating that it is a major factor in heart disease, depression, infectious diseases, digestive problems, auto-immune disorders, chronic pain and many forms of cancer. In simple terms, stress causes the body to lose its ability to regulate the inflammatory response.[13]

- The American Medical Association has noted that stress is the basic cause of more than 60 per cent of all human illness and disease[14]
- In the US, 75–90 per cent of primary care visits to physicians are for stress related problems[15]
- Emotional stress and trauma (emotional or physical) are a trigger for the growth of tumors[16]
- According to new Ohio State University research, stress fuels cancer by triggering a 'master switch'

At any one moment in time, the degree of stress may well be less than if we were facing a wild animal, but the unrelenting and complex interplay between stress, poor lifestyle habits and chronic disease is what is so depleting and harmful to our wellbeing today. Many of the symptoms of poor health and disease are both caused by and creating further stress.

Anxiety, addiction, work pressure, depression, tiredness, deficient nutrition, overeating, lack of exercise, poor breathing, anger, impatience, and all manner of chronic disease.

The human race today is characterized by chronic health problems because of a prevailing *normal* state of mind.

This creates a vicious cycle of diminishing wellbeing, symptomatic of a *normal* state of mind.

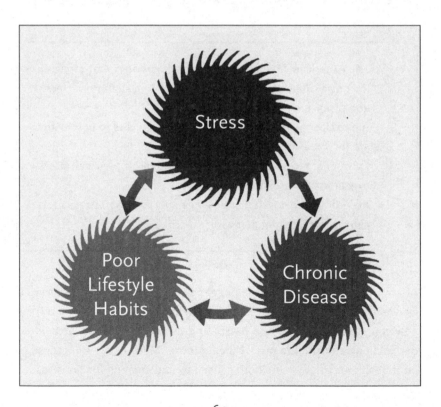

Please also note that with poor lifestyle habits come our destructive and unsustainable actions. So the above model explains the arising of the *normal* 'problem' trends that I spoke of before. At the root of the 'problem' lies our conditioned (stressed) quality of mind.

Stress is the silent stalker that carries no government health warning and is ubiquitously present in today's world

Notes

1. Harvard psychologists Matthew A. Killingsworth and Daniel T. Gilbert used a special 'track your happiness' iPhone app to gather research. The results showed that we spend at least half of our time thinking about something other than what we're engaged with, and this daydreaming doesn't make us happy. 'Wandering mind not a happy mind', *Harvard Gazette*, http://news.harvard.edu/gazette/story/2010/11/wandering-mind-not-a-happy-mind.
2. '2015 World Hunger and Poverty Facts and Statistics', www.worldhunger.org/articles/Learn/world%20hunger%20facts%202002.htm.
3. 'Child Poverty Facts and Figures', Child Poverty Action Group, www.cpag.org.uk/child-poverty-facts-and-figures.
4. '4 in 5 in USA Face Near-poverty, No Work ', USA Today, www.usatoday.com/story/money/business/2013/07/28/americans-poverty-no-work/2594203.
5. Colin D. Mathers and Dejan Loncar, 'Projections of Global Mortality and Burden of Disease from 2002 to 2030', http://journals.plos.org/plosmedicine/article?id=10.1371/journal.pmed.0030442.
6. Mark A. Hyman, 'Environmental Toxins, Obesity, and Diabetes: An Emerging Risk Factor', http://drhyman.com/downloads/Diabetes-and-Toxins.pdf.
7. Centers For Disease Control and Prevention.
8. Ruth S.M Chan and Jean Woo, 'Prevention of Overweight and Obesity: How Effective is the Current Public Health Approach', www.ncbi.nlm.nih.gov/pmc/articles/PMC2872299.
9. Quoted on Life Centre website, www.thelifecentre.com/therapies/yoga-therapy-at-islington.

10. By unconsciousness, I'm referring to the extent to which we're attached to our habitual thought patterns, beliefs, emotions and bodily sensations.
11. 'The Fight or Flight Response', Mind Body Soul Connection, https://holisticworld.co.uk/your_say.php?article_id=108.
12. It's really not possible to separate the body and the mind, since they are inextricably interwoven, wherein one impacts upon, and endlessly communicates with, the other. Because of this I will continue to refer to them as 'body-mind'.
13. The inflammatory response is, in simple terms, inflammation arising from bodily tissues being injured by such things as bacteria, trauma, toxins and heat. The damaged cells release chemicals which cause blood vessels to leak fluid into the tissues, causing swelling.
14. 'How Stress Affects the Body', Huffington Post, www.huffingtonpost.com/heartmath-llc/how-stress-affects-the-body_b_2422522.html.
15. Estimated by American Institute Of Stress.
16. 'Stress Linked to Cancer', Mercola.com, http://articles.mercola.com/sites/articles/archive/2010/02/04/stress-linked-to-cancer.aspx.

Summary Chapter 1

The Challenge and The Opportunity

Normal *vs* Natural

'Taming the Lake Monster' is a story which expresses the biggest problem that we face in life today — that our own mind is racing out of control. When the monster is allowed to behave in his normal, bothersome way, we are not very happy, and therefore not very healthy either, since happiness and health go hand in hand.

Herein lies a magnificent opportunity, since if we can tame our own lake monster, and we can, then we become the masters of our own health and happiness.

However, taming the lake monster is not easy, since we are so conditioned in the way that we think, speak and act — the *normal* state. The *normal* state is one in which we often breathe less fully than we need to, are perhaps careless with the needs of our body, and frequently experience stress. Yet, our *natural* state is to be vibrantly alive, neither stressed nor causing stress to others. The *natural* state is one in which we breathe efficiently, take care of the needs of our body and avoid stress.

Predominant Trends

If we look at the predominant trends of today, we can observe both a problem, and a corresponding opportunity –

The Problem – (*Normal* Quality Of Mind)

We frequently seem to be in resistance to nature's flow; many of us don't appear to be functioning as though we are part of the same human tribe. We increasingly seek to push the limits of this beautiful symphony called life, grabbing greedily at Mother Nature's resources; polluting the air and water one moment, then consuming it the next; and coveting all that we have not yet branded as ours.

The Opportunity – (*Natural* Quality Of Mind)

We have the possibility to Wake Up. Only we, the human race, can judiciously reflect upon our actions, override our normal, primal instincts and inclinations, and consciously decide upon a wiser course of action. We are the masters of our own wellbeing, and once we feel well, we can love all others like brothers and sisters, and take good care of our beautiful planet. In other words, we are able to flow with life just like the rest of nature.

Quality Of Mind

In simple terms, the quality of our life is determined by the quality of our mind – *normal* or *natural*. We have all been conditioned by our past, and the challenge that we face is to not be limited by the conditioned thinking which results. Given that most of us spend much of our time under the influence of a *normal* state of mind, there are certain recognizable tendencies – delegation of responsibility; a fear-based attitude; our attachment to a 'story', or voice, which runs unchecked; a tendency to suffer, due to our unwillingness to see and accept life as it actually is; and an array of needs and desires which captivate our imagination.

Stress

Stress is the inevitable outcome of being predominantly in our *normal* state of mind. Unfortunately, stress is so common and universally experienced that it has become like a modern-day plague. For many of us today, we are semi-permanently in a state of inner tension ('fight or flight'), which is compounded by our poor lifestyle habits, thus creating a vicious cycle of diminishing wellbeing and chronic disease. Inextricably woven into this cycle is the way in which we are impacting so negatively upon our earthly biosphere.

Chapter 2

The Solution
Wake Up and SOAR

What Can We Learn From Mother Nature?

In a word, *flow*.

Perhaps, deep down, all that we are truly seeking in today's fast-paced world, is calmness amidst the unending storm, a desire simply to flow gently with life.

My intention with this book, is to demonstrate that if we Wake Up and SOAR, then we too will learn how to flow with life. Through choosing where we focus our attention, breathing calmly, and therefore avoiding stress, we will experience our *natural* state of harmony. From here, we will be compassionate towards others, and mindful of our impact upon the planet.

The Nature of Nature

In observing the nature around us we can learn all we need to about ourselves, since Nature holds the mystical key to unlock the deepest truths within us. When we align ourselves with nature's flow, we experience our own essential nature – our *natural* quality of mind. Accordingly, the great Leonardo da Vinci said, 'Those who are inspired by a model other than nature, a mistress above all masters, are laboring in vain.'

Mother Nature's complete array of forms, including us humans, is made up of five elements. The essential element being space, or spirit, which underlies the other four – air, fire, water and earth. It is the flux within these five elements that creates life as it is. For example, if the Earth's plates (earth) were not moving towards or apart from each other, due to the cooling of the Earth (air and fire), none of the mountain ranges would exist, and the seas and oceans (water) of the earth would not be as they are. Just as the five elements express themselves in the outer climates of the world, so they describe the inner 'climates' of our bodies.

We humans would do well to observe Mother Nature's ways. No one element in her kingdom is more important than another, and each is humbly surrendered to the grand vision. There is never a rush, and all is flowing just as it needs to.

Mother Nature is a self-regulating web of life in a myriad of forms, where each part plays its role within the grand plan to maintain the health of the whole[1]

The Harmony of Mother Nature

All around us we see the endless unfolding of life in the multifarious forms of Mother Nature. Much of the time, this magnificent expression of life plays itself out with little or no drama. Then all at once we observe an event which might be quite dramatic, like a storm, and we see grand displays of energetic movement and transformation – gale-force winds and vast swathes of water cascading down a valley and uprooting trees.

Yet, moments later the winds die down, the water disappears and peace resumes. There may be some evidence of the storm in the form of debris, but other than this, harmony prevails. As I mentioned before, we can observe the same with animals, whereby they generally live harmoniously with one another, and then all at once there is confrontation, tension, and a fight or display of superiority arises. Shortly after, everything carries on as normal. In spite of her tendency for imbalance, Mother Nature is always rebalancing herself.

> **When Mother Nature becomes stressed,**
> **she has a magical way of releasing tension**

Cleansing and Renewal

Through Mother Nature's propensity for cleansing and renewal, the five elements are regulated and kept in balance: the seasons come and go, water levels rise and fall, planet Earth experiences natural cycles of warming and cooling, and we humans vacillate between balance and imbalance – healthy and sick, calm and stressed.

Even volcanoes, earthquakes, tsunamis and cyclones are all natural cleansing and renewal mechanisms, and whilst we humans term many of these phenomena 'natural disasters', none of the rest of nature is up in arms about them – they are simply accepted as a part of life.

There are clearly defined patterns and characteristics of this unceasing cleansing and renewal ritual of nature, in the form of impermanence, cycles and tension, each of which plays its part in the magical flow of life.

Impermanence

Nothing in life maintains the same form. Mother Nature is in a permanent state of evolution – moving from one state to another. We humans need to come to terms with this. Understanding this fact about life will help us to accept what we find unacceptable. It will help us to accept our faults so that we more easily move from a *normal*, troubled frame of mind, back to our *natural*, harmonious quality of mind.

It is impermanence which allows us to see evolution and growth. In just the same way that a mountain range develops through the earth's plates pushing together, so too do we humans grow through life's challenges.

**In order to grow, we must drop our resistance to what is arising,
in the knowledge that nothing lasts for long**

Cycles

Sometimes change is random, and at other times the five elements perform nature's cosmic dance according to cycles. For example, we see them in the form of the four seasons, as one phase transforms gradually, and sometimes not so gradually, into another.

If the moon were not performing an elliptical orbit around planet Earth, whilst Earth is orbiting the sun, there would be no such thing as the cycle of the moon. This cycle provides us with the magic of a full moon, which gradually shrinks and disappears to reveal Orion's Belt, incandescent against the night sky of a dark moon. Similarly, women have monthly cycles, and so too do we men, in our own unique way.[2]

The Indian monsoon is viewed in Ayurveda as the 'deep cleansing sweep' of Mother Nature, wherein weaknesses, or imbalances, are exposed, toxins are removed, and rest is invited – part of the grand cycle of ebbing and flowing. The fact that we humans have a daily cycle of sleeping and then being awake is what enables us to start each day fresh.

It's hard to know precisely the effect that we are having on the environment, but what seems clear is that if we fail to respect Mother Nature and her various cycles, we will imperil our own existence within her fragile biosphere.

Tension

It is quite natural for tension to arise in nature, just as it does within us humans. But generally speaking, the rest of Mother Nature's kingdom knows how to release tension far more effectively than we do. I spoke of dogs, cats and ducks before, but all animals know how to redress the balance when they become tense. It's natural that tension or 'hot spots' arise in the form of earthquakes, hurricanes, tsunamis and so on. Dramatic phenomena such as these may be devastating in human terms, but they are a part of nature's need to cleanse herself through releasing tension. They will arise, and they will then subside.

This is not to ignore or diminish the tragedy of such events, it is simply to say that life is an endless process of change. We may say that it is unfair,[3] but in the context of Mother Nature's vastness, it is merely what is happening in this moment — not good, not bad.

When through tectonic movement a volcano erupts and spews out vast quantities of molten ash and gases, the result is highly toxic for the surrounding biosphere. During the volcanic eruptions in Iceland in 2011, the toxic ash cloud was so expansive that it disrupted air travel for a number of weeks. Human life seems to be greatly disrupted, yet Mother Nature adapts, adjusts and accommodates according to her need for energetic transformation. We humans would do well to learn from this.

There are obvious hot spots in the human world — for example, the Middle East. However, unlike Mother Nature, we humans don't allow free expression. We seek to resist, and control, the actions of others when they have what we covet, or their actions don't suit our purposes.

Acceptance is, in my view, the noblest and most essential human quality. To accept a natural tragedy, or to accept the beliefs of others, or indeed, to humbly accept the distribution of Mother Nature's resources, requires our *natural* quality of mind.

> What causes human suffering, is our resistance to accepting something as it is. The more that we resist life as it actually is, the more we suffer. Dropping this resistance is therefore an opportunity for our evolution. Life is arising with an invitation for us to adapt, adjust and evolve. The more that we embrace this possibility, the more we flow with life.

The Flow Of Life

Everything which arises within Mother Nature's realm, has both a cause, and then in turn its own effect. Nothing acts in isolation of anything else, because everything is inextricably intertwined within the complex flow of life. Causality, or the law of cause and effect, is operating endlessly.

When the Indian monsoon delivers heavy rainfall, this creates a chain of events, or causes and effects: The groundwater level is higher than normal, which causes wells and boreholes to have more than enough water for the long dry season throughout much of India.

The effect of this is that farmers have plenty of food with which to feed their families, and an abundance of crops to sell at the markets. In turn this causes hundreds of millions of people to be able to meet their staple food needs, and perhaps even improve their diets.

Nature exudes the impression of being unflustered. Her myriad component parts are held in the embrace of an unspoken agreement – to participate in the game of life according to timeless and immutable laws. There is no rush, no waste and everything flows effortlessly.

The Healing Arts

The healing arts are ancient practices which were created to optimize health and happiness, and prevent human suffering and sickness. They include such practices as yoga, meditation, homeopathy, Ayurveda, Tai chi, Chinese medicine and Zen shiatsu, which all have their roots in Mother Nature's teachings. These great healing systems recognized that good health requires the harmonious balance of the five elements.

Because these ancient bodies of wisdom are so grounded in the wisdom of Mother Nature, they represent a beautiful and potent example of what we can learn from her. Not surprisingly perhaps, when they are practiced in their fullest expression, they are profound vehicles for transformation. They cause us to be progressively more attentive to the depth of our being. In other words, they invite us to calm our mind and return to our *natural* state.

Without learning to do this, the human experience is like a car at night without headlights – aimless, unfulfilling and potentially quite damaging.

They have therefore made it their craft to examine and explain the ways in which we humans can redress our imbalances, in order to relax our bodies, calm our minds and attune with our spirit.

The great sages, such as Gautama Siddhartha (the pre-enlightened Buddha), practiced rigorous self-discipline. The purpose of this was to develop great focus and concentration, and therefore invite their *natural* quality of mind. But they also observed the nature around them with the same non-judgmental awareness. They intuited much about the effortless flow of life, and saw just how surrendered animals, plants and rocks were to the grand plan. They observed how the animals moved and stretched, effortlessly taking care of the physical needs of their bodies, and hence yoga postures, asanas, have animal names.

Through their ability to calm their minds, these sages were also able to tap into ageless wisdom. They therefore had great knowledge about the workings of the human body, including its various systems – endocrine, respiratory, cardiovascular, immune and so on. Before science was 'science' as we know it today, it was simply non-judgmental observation.

Interestingly, the methodology of the ancient mystics and today's great scientists are remarkably similar. In fact, I've noticed that a number of modern meditation teachers and scientists have described the path of meditation as a form of 'scientific investigation', using very specific procedures that lead to recognizable and predictable results.

What we are witnessing with increasing regularity is just how profoundly modern science is validating so much of ancient wisdom. For example, Youngey Mingyur Rinpoche, a Buddhist monk, has been a test subject for some of the most cutting-edge neurological studies. Through understanding how the mind transforms the brain, he came to realize that contemporary scientific theory and his meditation practices were aligned.

Yoga and meditation are truly coming of age in the west, and there are a burgeoning number of books, posts and articles across the internet which espouse the medical research into the benefits of these practices. There are, of course, some articles and books which speak of potential negative effects, but this is the case with any wellbeing or healing system where insufficient consideration is given to the particular needs of an individual.

In the main, studies conclusively show that yoga and meditation can increase oxygen delivery and blood flow, keep your muscles and joints strong and flexible, as well as improve your attention, concentration and short-term memory.

Traditionally, meditation begins with looking inwards and concentrating your attention on just one thing – your breathing, or perhaps a mantra (the repetition of Sanskrit words). With practice, this can yield single-pointed focus, or a high degree of concentration. This is the same process as 'mindfulness' in Buddhism, where you focus your attention on the emotions, thoughts and sensations with non-judgmental awareness.

Apart from the obvious physical benefits, the essential purpose of these ancient systems is that you calm your mind and return to your *natural* state, so that you remember how to flow effortlessly like Mother Nature.

'Wake Up and SOAR'

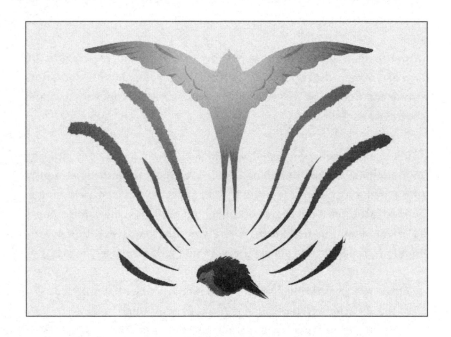

There is a simple way to ensure that you are in your *natural* state, rather than a *normal* state – Wake Up and SOAR. This is a simple tool which allows you to move from the *normal* state to your *natural* state whenever you choose to.

Wake Up and SOAR is the essential tool for loving your life

You will notice that this has two parts to it – Wake Up, and SOAR.

Wake Up

First you have to realize that your lake monster is thrashing about, and you are frequently giving your attention to him. Like a pool cleaner, your mind is sucking up the debris around its nozzle.

When you are held hostage by your mind in this way, your attention is not here in this present moment. Instead, you are distracted by your story – the inner dialogue of your mind.

In the story of the lake monster, it was the voice from the sky which woke the lake up – 'One day a loud and resonant voice came from the sky and spoke directly to the lake ...'

Think of it like this. A friend comes to your home and asks if you are there. Your partner, flatmate or whoever, calls to you but hears no reply, and therefore tells your friend that you're not at home at the moment.

The first step then, is that you Wake Up to the realization that you're not at home, because your lake monster is captivating your attention. Through this realization, you are magically teleported back home.

However, once you begin this little practice of Waking Up, you will see that it happens rather frequently. In other words, you will see that you are endlessly not at home – probably a lot more than you *are* at home.

On the next page, there are some questions that I'd like you to read. These are intended to help you to realize just how often you are in your *normal* state of mind.

- Are you aware of those things that you do much faster than you need to – for example racing to brush your teeth, or to get ready in the morning?
- Are you generally thinking about events in the future, because they are more exciting than the present reality?
- Are you aware of your bodily sensations – for example the difference between the sensation of stretching gently, compared with the sharper pain of stretching too far?
- Do you notice taking a deep breath when you are challenged?
- Can you easily tell the difference between thirst and hunger, when you are slightly dehydrated?
- Can you easily sense what you truly want? In other words, can you tell the difference between what you think you want, and what you need, or truly desire, in any given moment?
- Are you aware of when you are breathing easily and effortlessly?
- How easy is it for you to accept what arises when it is counter to what you actually want?
- Can you surrender your will when you realize the greater good in doing so?
- Do you know how to relax when you most need to?
- Are you aware of the deep, still silence that resides permanently within your being?

Awakening

When you are in your *normal* state of mind, you can't choose to be in your *natural* state of mind. You first have to Wake Up. There are three possible ways in which you can awaken –

1. Force of circumstances can stimulate your awakening

If you're free climbing a sheer rock face, then you'd better be fully awake and present to this moment, otherwise you risk plummeting to your death. Your awakening is therefore stimulated by the particular circumstances that you are in. Equally, this might also be when you are on stage performing, or perhaps scuba diving underwater.

2. You can awaken by chance

The most common way for us to awaken is by chance. By which I mean that there is no apparent reason why you should awaken in the particular moment that you do. You might be walking along the road, and suddenly realize that for the last few moments you were completely lost in thought, and oblivious to what was going on around you.

3. You can invite awakening through practices such as SOAR

This means that you're sufficiently aware of how often you're lost in thought that you've made an earnest commitment to no longer be incessantly distracted by your lake monster. Because of this, you invite your own awakening through your clarity of intention. It's my hope that after reading this book, this will be the case for you.

SOAR

The second step then, is about being at home in your *natural* state. Once you've Woken Up, it's as though time stops, and you have the opportunity to climb into the 'space' which is created. So SOAR is a tool which allows you to enter that gap, and then sit there quietly, amidst the stillness.

SOAR is an acronym, which stands for –

S – Slow down (sit down and close your eyes if possible)

O – Observe inwardly and connect with your breath

A – Accept all that is arising without judgment or resistance

R – Relax deeply and sense your inner peace of being

Each of these letters therefore represents one part of a four-step sequence that will allow you to return to, or maintain, your calm, *natural* state. SOAR is a tool of introspection which can be applied to any situation in life, once you've Woken Up. On awakening, you automatically recognize the possibility to remain in the space of calm, which is there beyond your busy mind. But, rest assured, the mind will keep knocking at the door of your quiet sanctuary.

So, looking at the three ways in which you can awaken, described overleaf, we have the three uses for the tool SOAR –

1   It can be used when force of circumstances stimulate your awakening – as well as free climbing, this might also happen if you've awoken in a moment when you are mentally and emotionally 'triggered', and you wish to stay calm.

2   It can be used when you awaken by chance and want to stay more focused on what you're doing – for example, whilst at work on a Friday afternoon at 4pm, and your mind is wandering towards your evening plans.

3   It can be used as a practice to enter your *natural* state (which will also invite awakening more frequently) – for example, to aid you in falling asleep at night, since when your mind is calm the need for sleep takes over.

The intention with SOAR is that you stop giving attention to the outer world that you perceive through your senses – sight, sound, smell, touch and taste; and instead, you begin to notice what is there underneath your busy mind. Choosing to not give attention to your busy mind allows you to experience the vast well of stillness which is already there at the source of your being. And if you're free climbing, emotionally triggered, struggling to stay focused, or wishing to fall asleep at night, then this is extremely beneficial and pleasant. This is why I have referred to it as 'coming home'.

So let's check this out practically. If you are not already sitting down, please do so now, and then read and follow the instructions in the next paragraph. I invite you to read and follow the instructions a few times until you have a clear sense of your own experience – whatever that might be.

Close your eyes for a moment and observe what is going on inside. Simply pay attention to what is arising. Ignore everything that is happening outside of you, and focus all of your attention inwards.

Have you started to sense what I spoke of a moment ago? Can you see what makes it hard for you to experience your sense of inner peace?

Your thoughts are endlessly arising. They just keep coming. Your lake monster is thrashing about, and you are giving him a lot of your attention. Sometimes your thoughts are a stream of related ideas or images, and at other times they spring forth randomly and are not linked at all.

Perhaps some of you had a sense of calmness, and others of you none at all. Either way, it's fine. What's really important is that you see what stands in your way, before you can do anything about it. The clearer you see the impediment, the easier it will be to deal with it.

In the moment you realize that you are in some way resisting life by attaching to an unsolicited thought, or a disturbing emotion, and you choose to not continue that thought, or to not give attention to that emotion or sensation, you set yourself free.

So to be clear, your thoughts are not the problem. The problem is that, to a greater or lesser extent, you are giving them your attention. If you are choosing to 'have' a thought, then there's no problem. But what happens most of the time is that thoughts are arising for no particular reason, and 'your attention is seduced by them'. You are so used to giving your thoughts, emotions and bodily sensations your undivided attention that this feels normal.

Maybe you can begin to sense that so long as you allow your thoughts to be the master of your attention, you cannot be the master of your own wellbeing?

The tool SOAR is all about interrupting your habitual pattern of giving your attention to unsolicited thoughts, and instead choosing where you direct your attention (with a laser-like focus).

The thoughts that you unconsciously give your attention to (because you are in a *normal* frame of mind) are like passing clouds. They have every right to be there, but that doesn't mean that you have to keep climbing aboard them. Let them pass. Allow them to float by, leaving you calm and undistracted.

Is it hard for most of us to sense our inner peace?

Yes. But you can now see why this is. You are so busy attending to every thought that there is no possibility for you to sense what is already there, underneath:

> *'Deep within the lake everything was serene and perfect, yet the lake was full of sadness. No one had ever seen her true beauty, or the magical crystals in all their glory, since the surface waters of the lake were inhabited by a monster who believed that he was the ruler of this watery kingdom.'*

The lake monster is not at fault, he is just doing what he has always done. You have to show him that he's not the boss, so that he can also relax. Liberation from your lake monster requires that you tame him, and this requires heartfelt desire and vigilance. Anything less, and you will quickly lose interest in practicing SOAR.

But isn't it true that anything worth having requires at least a little effort? Are relationships plain sailing? Is your job or daily activity a breeze? Is mastering anything easy for that matter? No, of course not. We all know that success in any sphere of life requires concerted effort. This journey together is not going to be without effort. But I can promise you that the rewards are beyond measure. I shall say more about this in just a moment.

So, let's try again. I'm going to ask you to close your eyes again, therefore you'll need to read the instructions overleaf first. I'm also going to ask you to do this exercise in the following way:

- Read Step 1, follow the instructions, and then open your eyes
- Read Step 2, then do steps 1 and 2 together (then open your eyes)
- Read Step 3, then do steps 1, 2 and 3 together (then open your eyes)
- Read Step 4, then do steps 1, 2, 3 and 4 together (then open your eyes)

You might need to open your eyes a few times to re-read the instructions. That's fine.

Step 1: Slow down[4] – If you are not already seated, please sit down now. Check that your back is straight, but without tension. Close your eyes. Take a moment to adjust your position so that you are as comfortable as possible.

Step 2: Observe inwardly – Focus your attention inwards, becoming aware of your breathing. (You can either sense the breath in your belly, or at the tip of your nose). Make sure that your breathing is slow, rhythmical and effortless. (Try doing this for approximately one minute.)

Step 3: Accept all that is arising – As you focus on your breathing, let your thoughts flow without engaging with them. Simply choose not to touch them as they arise, and stay more interested in your breathing. If you find yourself momentarily lost in thought, bring your attention back to your breathing (keep doing this until it becomes more effortless).

Step 4: Relax deeply – As you feel yourself becoming more relaxed, begin to sense what is there underneath the breath, before the thoughts. Can you sense an inner ease, a stillness, an expansiveness?

(Please don't try to sense something, just allow what is there to be there, and notice without judgment or coming to any conclusions.)

Some of you might still be feeling unsure as to what this is all about; others of you are perhaps able to glimpse what is there beyond the arising of thoughts; and if you are already feeling quite calm through this process, then fine. But in truth, the most important thing right now is that you see just how busy your mind is when you are in a *normal* state.

The 'Pot of Gold'

You, me, all of us, have been searching for something. Knowingly, or unknowingly, we have been looking for an answer, some salvation, a quick fix to this thing called life. Yet, the joke of it all, is that what we've truly been seeking, is precisely who we already are, at depth. As I said in the introduction:

> *'In short, the outer human quest is nothing other than our deep desire to journey inwards back to our Source, disguised as something apparently more stimulating.'*

So how do you resolve this paradox?

Keep coming home to your *natural* state:

Wake Up and SOAR

We will keep practicing SOAR throughout the book, and I am confident that if you really apply yourself to the practice, you will begin to sense a deep, inner wellbeing that is permanent, and independent of whatever else is going on. But to facilitate this, I want to spell out exactly what I think you can gain from the practice, in the hope that it will inspire you to truly apply yourself:

- When your mind is calm, you sense the depth of your being – you discover that safe, private place at the core of your being, where you are able to rest, and feel calm and contented.
- This is what causes you to feel vibrantly alive – it's like having deep roots connected to the source of your being.
- From here, you are able to focus your attention like a laser beam because your mind is quiet – in other words, you are able to give your full, undivided attention to whatever or whomever you choose.

- Because your life force is now focused like a beam of light, you enliven whatever you give your attention to – you become a beacon of light for others, 'infecting' them with your positive vibration.

Whilst it's important to practice SOAR, what I really encourage you to focus on are the results of the practice, as mentioned above – beginning with your sense of inner calm and contentment.

Therefore the intention of the book is that you learn this practice so that you become familiar with your inner resting place. This is actually not a 'place', it's who you really are – the essence of you. When you 'get past' your busy mind, you realize that underneath it all, you are actually incredibly well, and always have been. You are then able to increasingly live your life from here – your *natural* quality of mind.

This book is not meant to be theoretical. It's intended to be a practical guide that you can use directly in your everyday life. The message here is profoundly simple. But, as I said before, quieting the *normal* state of mind is a tricky business. Your conditioning is hard-wired into your subconscious mind, and the habits that march to the beat of this drum have incredible momentum.

Therefore, there are really two things that stand between you and a life of peace, joy and abundant love –

- The first is the momentum of your lake monster – the persistent thoughts which distract you so much that you forget to Wake Up.
- The second is your resolve – your commitment to SOAR, and to keep SOARing whenever you remember.

This is why it's so important that you commit to the practice. It's a very simple practice, but your lake monster is tricky and seductive. I believe that we all need guidance and support in life.

If the greatest athletes on Earth have coaches and trainers to support them in excelling in their chosen field, then why wouldn't you and I need support when it comes to taking charge of our lives?

My intention is that the journey of the book ignites your inner thirst for awakening so strongly that using and applying the tools becomes inevitable. However, if your desire for taking charge of your health and happiness is not sincere, then the book will be of little good.

Notes

1.   Inspired by the Gaia hypothesis of Dr James Lovelock.
2.   It's known that men's testosterone levels are cyclical just as women's hormones are, though the exact nature of this is not well understood.
3.   As I write these words, we are in the immediate aftermath of the Nepalese earthquake (late April 2015). Six of Ashiyana's staff are Nepalese, and at this moment we are engaged in a fund-raising program to help them and their families to rebuild their homes and lives.
4.   The first step, 'Slow down', becomes all the more relevant when you are busy with, or rushing to do, something. In this *normal* situation, if the urge to SOAR arises – because you Wake Up, then first slow down in whatever you're doing, and if possible sit down and close your eyes.

Summary Chapter 2

The Solution
Wake Up and SOAR

Learning from Mother Nature

At the depth of our being, we are in harmony with Mother Nature – this is our *natural* state. We need to keep recognizing how effortlessly Mother Nature goes about her daily tasks, and seek to replicate this in our own lives.

Mother Nature reveals the secret to calming our lake monster – she always returns to her default setting of ease and equanimity through a natural process of cleansing and renewal. This helps us to accept our own human tendency to vacillate between *normal* and *natural* qualities of mind.

Just like Mother Nature, every part of our being is interconnected with all other parts, so when one organ is out of balance, our whole system is involved in the re-balancing process.

Mother Nature teaches us that co-operation, not competition, is the key to flourishing. We need to keep realizing how totally in harmony the rest of nature is. Life is an invitation for us to accept whatever is arising without resistance – once we are calm, we can then adapt, adjust and evolve. The more that we embrace this possibility, the more that we flow with life

The Healing Arts

The healing arts are ancient practices which were created to optimize health and happiness, and prevent human suffering and sickness. Because these ancient bodies of wisdom are so grounded in the wisdom of Mother Nature, they represent a beautiful and potent example of what we can learn from her. Not surprisingly perhaps, when they are practiced in their fullest expression, they are profound vehicles for transformation.

Wake Up and SOAR

This is a simple but very potent tool which allows you to move from the *normal* state to your *natural* state at will.

Wake Up – First you have to realize that your lake monster is thrashing about, and you are frequently giving your attention to him. You are distracted by your story – the inner dialogue of your mind.

SOAR

S – Slow down (sit down and close your eyes if possible)
O – Observe inwardly and connect with your breath
A – Accept all that is arising without judgment or resistance
R – Relax deeply and sense your inner peace of being

If you apply yourself to the practice you will begin to sense a deep, inner wellbeing that is independent of whatever else is going on.

The 'Pot of Gold'

When your mind is calm, you sense the depth of your being.
This is what causes you to feel vibrantly alive.
From here, you are able to focus your attention like a laser beam .
Because your life force is now focused like a beam of light, you enliven whatever you give your attention to.

As I mentioned in the introduction, since *normal* and *natural* are so fundamental to the message, I will continually refer to them throughout the rest of the book. My intention is that each time you see these words you take a moment to reflect on your own quality of mind. In other words, you use these as prompts to Wake Up and SOAR.

Chapter 3

The Power Of Acceptance

It's About Surrender

We've identified the 'problem' – our tendency to be in a *normal* state of mind. I've offered the 'solution' – Wake Up and SOAR – a tool which enables you to return to your *natural* quality of mind at will.

This chapter offers a deeper understanding of the power contained within SOAR. When you truly learn to accept yourself, just as you are, you magically transform your life experience.

SOAR is really about surrender. Not in the sense of giving up in battle, but in the sense of accepting whatever you are experiencing in your mind, emotions and body. This means allowing thoughts to float by which you don't want to engage with, without resisting them; and if you have engaged with a thought that you have not 'chosen' to have, you can simply drop it at will.

With surrender, there is no need to hide anything, and you are therefore willing to show yourself just as you are. You know how this feels. I know you do.

How do I know?

I know, because we've all had this experience of feeling utterly safe. It might be with a loved one, or perhaps when you are walking alone in nature. The circumstances are not important. What is important is that you know what it is like to be naked before life. This is real freedom. The freedom to be 100 per cent yourself, no editing, and no finessing. Just you – ALL of you!

The magnificent possibility to accept all that arises, is the doorway to a peaceful quality of mind, and therefore mastery over your mind. This quality of acceptance invites you into the here and now – it is the essence of your *natural* state.

Bob Marley sang about this – 'Emancipate yourselves from mental slavery, none but ourselves can free our minds.' Through detaching from what you are not intentionally giving your attention to, you create space in your being, within which all is allowed, nothing is resisted, and surrendered acceptance prevails.

So acceptance is not passive. It is having the intention to let go of thoughts that you are not really interested in giving your attention to. You are accepting that they are there, but you are choosing to not give them your attention. First you notice the thought (Wake Up). Then you choose to stay calm and to neither resist, nor touch, the thought that is arising (SOAR).

As I said before:

> *'In the moment you realize that you are in some way resisting life by attaching to an unsolicited thought, a disturbing emotion or a bodily sensation, and you choose to not continue that thought, or to not give attention to that emotion or sensation, you set yourself free.'*

Please remind yourself what this feels like –

S – Slow down (sit down and close your eyes if possible)

O – Observe inwardly and connect with your breath

A – Accept all that is arising without judgment or resistance

R – Relax deeply and sense your inner peace of being

With surrendered acceptance your energy field is expanded, and you create inner space. With spaciousness, you give yourself the possibility consciously to choose where you put your attention, and therefore focus your life force – you become the master of your life experience, and you have razor-sharp concentration.

Your quality of mind determines how you feel about, and deal with, a situation. At times of difficulty, you will often become contracted – *normal* state. Your emotional body (that aspect of your being which allows you to experience desires, feelings and emotions) has fallen prey to fear, anxiety, anger, confusion and so on, which causes a physical contraction and varying degrees of stress.

Maybe you sense that sometimes you dread the arising of life's challenges?

But life simply arises, *it just is*.

Through surrendered acceptance, you return to your *natural* state, so that you avoid mental, emotional and physical tension. The prevailing spaciousness allows you to feel calm.

In the *natural* state, your expanded consciousness puts you in touch with universal wisdom. So before you make any important decisions, SOAR. This is a mature way of approaching life, because when you are calm, there is no resistance. From here, you will have the wisdom to determine whether you can do something about a situation or not.

If you realize that you are able to change the circumstances in which you find yourself, then with spaciousness you sense the appropriate action, knowing that whatever you say or do will be benign and therefore fitting.

If, however, you realize that there is really nothing that you can do to change or moderate the situation that you are in, and you need to simply accept the circumstances, then through surrender you stay calm and detached.

Spaciousness is deeply connected with breathing, and breathing is our most essential connection with Mother Nature. If you take a few full, deep breaths, observing the way in which this animates your belly, ribs and chest, you cannot help but feel calm and relaxed. When you sense resistance, and you set it free by consciously breathing in this way, it's as if you 're-boot your system', and bring everything back into balance.

> *'We humans are designed to flow, just like the seasons. Even our breath flows like the tide – when we breathe in we draw in life force, or 'prana', and when we breathe out we let go of tension, tiredness and toxins.'*

Accept Yourself

One of the many things that Satyananda has helped me to see is that the greatest irritation which we face is not the arising of our human emotions, but the way in which we chastise ourselves for them. We set ourselves up for a fall by comparing our programed images of how we think we should be with how we actually are.

This is destined to create inner tension, and therefore suffering. We are unconsciously punishing ourselves for being human and for having emotions – 'I shouldn't become angry', 'I should have more patience', 'It's wrong to feel like this', and so on.

> *Can you think of a situation in the recent past where you've been chastising yourself for the way that you have reacted to, or felt about, something? Maybe you can also sense how this has perhaps limited you in some way, and stopped you from being all that you are – 100 per cent You?*

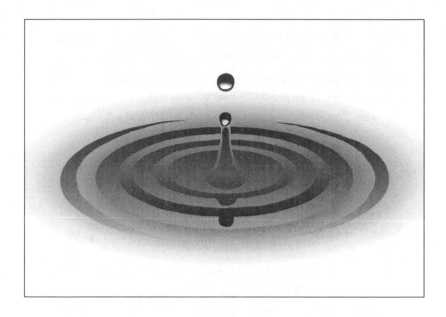

Life invites us to grow, not to criticize ourselves. Yet we don't give our human traits the space to arise and pass by without resistance, as a storm or an earthquake does in nature. Instead we judge our brief moments of humanness very harshly, and therefore attempt to suppress them, creating tension. As any observer of life knows, when you suppress something you give it power — you literally enliven it with your life force.

Experiencing feelings and bodily sensations because of our human emotions is fine, and not the problem. The problem arises through our judgments about, and therefore resistance to, these feelings. This creates our suffering. It is rather comical when you see it this way. It's as though we are standing in moral judgment of life itself — 'According to my filter, things shouldn't be this way. Life is making a mistake here!'

We are not designed to be perfect. There is no perfection. Nature is perfect in its imperfection. So the trick is not to beat yourself up, but rather to let go of the thoughts that disturb you. When you accept yourself, you will be able to accept all others, and all else. Some pain is inevitable, but suffering is optional.

'You Are Ok As You Are'

Let me exemplify this by recounting a Skype conversation that I had with Satyananda recently.

'You are ok as you are.' These are the words that Satyananda told me over and over again. I had heard him say this to me and to others, many times before, and in various different ways. But today was different.

This had been one of the most challenging periods of my life, and yet, paradoxically, also one of the most exciting. I was suffering with great sadness about my girlfriend, or ex-girlfriend. I wasn't sure which she was. At the same time, it looked like the book that I was writing (this book) was going to be published. This was an important book for me, since it was part of a bigger vision that was perhaps going to be the most exciting creation of my life.

I called Satyananda on Skype from my room at Ashiyana in Goa. He made a joke about the fact that I was wearing a vest and shorts, and he was wrapped up in layers of clothes, topped by his poncho. Satyananda is from Uruguay, but lives in England. With his long hair and beard he is truly South American in appearance, especially when adorned with a poncho and drinking his mate tea. He looked at me with his gentle but profound gaze, and asked me how I was.

'I'm feeling sad,' I replied.

'You remember that I was with Cristina¹ over the summer. She had the daughter, and we were living together in a small house with one bedroom. I was totally in love for the first few weeks, and then after a while it was too much for me. I needed space, and then started to close down. My heart was closing. I couldn't show her love anymore. I needed to get away. I left Brazil at the end of August. This is a repeating pattern for me. Whenever things become difficult, I run away.'

Satyananda paused and replied, 'Well I don't see it that way. It's normal to feel pressure in a relationship. It's normal to want to be alone, to not sleep in the same bed, and to not want to be part of the plans of another. You are not hurting anyone. You have the right to run away. That was right for you in that moment. You were being guided. You are always being guided. You are ok as you are. Never again think that you're not ok, that you've got to change.'

With these words, I relaxed. I knew deep inside me that what he was saying was true. Chastising myself for having run away and hurt her was a waste of time, and was also not respecting the fact that life was guiding me. Something within me had known that it was not right for me to be with Cristina.

This exchange helped me to understand more deeply the meaning of 'accept yourself'. I realized that:

Nothing needs to change. Nothing is wrong.
I am perfect as I am.

I am aware that the words above are easily misunderstood. So let me be completely clear. I am not suggesting that I couldn't have behaved in a more loving and compassionate way with Cristina, particularly towards the end. My point is this: I had the right to feel overwhelmed; and in truth life was guiding me wisely.

How I dealt with the situation, being closed and incommunicative, and then feeling bad about this, was a symptom of my *normal* state of mind. In this state, I was having thoughts, and perhaps saying and doing things, which were simply not me 'at my best'. (I'm sure that you can relate to this.) The resolution to this was, and is, not to beat myself up, but rather to relax and come back to my *natural* quality of mind. From here, I can sense what is best for me to say and do – and this allows me to be 'at my best'.

So accepting yourself means you recognize that nothing about you, fundamentally, needs to change. Rather it's your quality of mind which needs addressing. After all, your personality is nothing more than an expression of your quality of mind.

This then addresses the whole issue of getting better – 'I should be better', 'I need to improve', 'I am not worthy of this, that or the other', and so on ...

Yes, we can all improve. But what does this actually mean? If you are in your *normal* frame of mind, and you chastise yourself, or even gently reprimand yourself for what you've thought, said or done, you are simply fighting fire with fire.

> You don't need to improve. You don't need to get better. You don't need to do anything in fact, until you have first come home to your safe resting place within.

Just accept yourself exactly as you are – Wake Up and SOAR – and all will become clear, or, at least, it will become clearer.

I therefore invite you to consider that the words written below are true for you also. Please repeat these words aloud a few times. Then close your eyes, and sense how you feel as the vibration of these words washes over you.

Nothing needs to change. Nothing is wrong.
I am perfect as I am.

Be Guided By Life

To solve any 'problem', you need to adjust the lens through which you're seeing the problem. In other words, what you perceive to be the 'problem' is not actually the problem. It's the way that you're 'seeing' the situation (through the lens of a contracted, *normal* state of mind) that is the problem.

So, always come home first – Wake Up and SOAR – before you come to any decisions or conclusions about what does, or does not, need to be done.

**The *normal* state of mind cannot solve the
'problems' created by the same state of mind.
Only the *natural* quality of mind can achieve this.**

I hope that this is clear, because it is so important to understand. This realization simplifies life beyond anything imaginable. It's really not helpful to beat yourself up, or endlessly criticize others. You simply need to come home to your *natural* quality of mind, because from here, calmness prevails and you therefore see things clearly.

Growth, or being guided by life, in the sense that I mean it, is the alchemical process that arises when you allow life to transform something within your being. In returning to your *natural* quality of mind, you surrender your rigid ego mind to the cleansing ways of Mother Nature, and you allow her to reset you.

It is like a re-calibration, or a shift in perspective which life takes care of, and not one that you can control. Therefore, you don't have to try to grow. What you can do is be aware of what causes your suffering, and learn to accept it.

If you can find peace with what disturbs you, you disempower it by ceasing to give it your attention, your life force. Once you've shown that a particular belief, person or situation no longer troubles you, life stops presenting you with that challenge. At least, this has been my experience.

So being guided by life means accepting everything as though you had asked for it. This way, nothing has control over you or your emotions.

Everything in life is energy vibrating, so be aware of your vibration. Sense how your habitual thoughts and beliefs are creating your vibration, and thence attracting your life towards you. (Chapter 4 is devoted to this subject.) When you accept life as it is, rather than sit in judgment of it, you open yourself to wise guidance from within.

As Satyananda said, 'You are always being guided.' Through acceptance, you access your *natural* quality of mind, and your inner eyes see clearly. From here, you recognize how life is guiding you. When you are calm, and your lake monster is tamed, you will intuit what to say and do. You won't need to stress, worry or struggle over decisions. An infinite field of creative wisdom is at play – you step aside with your *normal*, contracted mind, and allow your inner wisdom to guide you.

All wise teachings invite this melting into surrendered acceptance. Indeed, it is the 'fast track to peace and wellbeing', since it bypasses the need for a path, a practice or any form of teacher or teaching – it simply transports you to the end goal directly.

If you behave as though whatever arises is precisely what you have asked for, then you will magically transform your life.

Resisting Others

Whatever you don't accept in yourself, you will tend to resist outside of you. So when you find something unacceptable 'out there', you can be sure that it is mirroring something within you that has not been accepted by you. Observe nature and see how she eagerly finds ease, the path of least resistance.

Your path of least resistance is to accept everything that arises within you with compassion, realizing that it is a part of you. It has the right to be there, and indeed, is there for a reason. When you fully accept yourself, you will naturally accept others too.

I have found this more and more to be the case. Even though my first reaction towards someone might be judgmental, after a moment or two I will often realize that what is upsetting me about them is reflecting something about me. When I remember that 'I'm ok', compassion for others naturally arises.

Please check this out for yourself. Think of a situation when you have been upset with someone. Allow yourself to feel the upset, the raised heartbeat and the tension in your belly.

Now Wake Up and SOAR.

'Stand back' from the situation, recognizing that you can impassively observe what is arising, and SOAR –

S – Slow down (sit down and close your eyes if possible)

O – Observe inwardly and connect with your breath

A – Accept all that is arising without judgment or resistance

R – Relax deeply and sense your inner peace of being

How do you feel towards this person now?

This is a virtuous circle, because learning to have compassion for others will also help you to accept yourself as you are, with all of your faults and rough edges.

Letting Go

When spaciousness prevails, you free your heart from hatred, and your mind from worries. Hatred and worry stem from fear, and since there is ample space within you for fear to flow and dissipate, you 'let it go'. Letting go requires clarity and courage – clarity to dispassionately observe fear when it arises, and courage to not resist it. Behind the fear there is actually nothing there, just memories that you have attached to.

Any resistance within your body-mind ultimately stems from fear – fear of the unknown, fear of intimacy, fear of being seen, fear of being wrong, fear of looking foolish, fear of hurting someone, and so on.

My conversation with Satyananda is a case in point. I had been fearful of expressing my vulnerability and inner struggle with my ex-girlfriend. I hope that when faced with this same scenario again, I will find the courage to speak about my feelings more openly. But it's important that I don't feel guilty about ideas of wrong-doing, which arise from a *normal* state of mind.

In today's world, feelings of guilt, shame and inadequacy are so prevalent, and we find any opportunity to beat ourselves up – 'I should be better', 'I need to improve', 'I am not worthy of this, that or the other'.

It was clear from my dialogue with Satyananda that I too was full of such feelings:

'This is a repeating pattern for me. Whenever things become difficult, I run away.'

Whilst I can see that the difficulty I had in communicating my feelings clearly to Cristina caused the relationship to become such a struggle for me, feeling guilty was of no help whatsoever. The guilt only caused tension within my body and mind. The way for me to learn and grow was to let go of my guilt and self-judgment.

In my view, letting go doesn't stand in the way of growth. In fact, it creates the possibility for it. Sometimes we need to understand clearly what has gone on in a situation, other times not. But what will always benefit a situation is taking space, breathing, and allowing equanimity to prevail. Every situation in life is unique, and that's why a calm mind is so key for determining the best course of action.

Satyananda's point wasn't that I had nothing to learn from my suffering. He was inviting me to see that I was not allowing vulnerability in myself, and was therefore not comfortable in showing this part of myself to Cristina. He was helping me to understand the situation, so that I would be at peace with it.

Is it easy for me to be vulnerable with those I love, or indeed with myself?

Certainly not always. But when I remember to embrace the gift of acceptance (SOAR), fear dissipates and I feel calm. When I accept that

I have conditioned thoughts and emotions, I can easily choose not to touch them. From here, I can see the best way to speak or act.

There is no diet, no tincture and no magical panacea that will tackle the universal quest for happiness and wellbeing half as efficaciously as surrendered acceptance

The 10 Mantras (Mini-meditations)

A mantra is a word or sound that is repeated in order to aid concentration when meditating.

Whist I was writing the book, certain phrases kept coming to mind. I see these phrases, or mantras, as life's support and guidance for my journey. When I fail to embrace them, I seem to endlessly attract the same situations into my life. I therefore invite you to read the following section and see which of these mantras might support you in navigating the pathway of your life more serenely.

If you look closely at the list below, you will sense that they have a common root – they each originate from, and point towards, your *natural* quality of mind. In other words, they are prompts for awakening and therefore developing a calm quality of mind.

I find that, according to a given situation, I will remember one of them, and that will trigger my awakening. For example, if I am being miserly, I will spontaneously remember the third realization, and my inner tension will subside.

1   Be Positive and Open to Opportunities

2   Nurture Honesty and Integrity

3   Give More and Expect Less

4   Follow the Middle Path

5   Develop Trust in Life

6   Nurture Flexibility

7   Have Gratitude

8   Laugh Easily

9   Be Patient

10 Love

As you read the following pages, take your time, and SOAR intermittently as you read.

I invite you to join me in closing your eyes. Just allow whatever arises to float by. Don't attach to it. Stay here. Find your breathing more interesting than the arising thoughts and sensations. Keep gently accepting that whatever is happening is fine. Don't resist it, but don't be seduced by it either.

1. Be Positive and Open to Opportunities

Viewing life positively or negatively is usually a habit. Like all habits, momentum is created, which means that when you are in a *normal* state, you are often swept along in habitual, reactive patterns. So being positive is not about 'trying to be nice', or 'doing what someone else wants', but rather expanding the lens through which you see the world.

A positive mindset is something that needs to be cultivated, so when you see yourself contracting and reacting, take a breath or two, and choose instead to focus on the positive that is there. I believe that every situation has a positive side to it, even if only that you sense how challenging your predicament is, and you develop resolve. I have constantly found in my life, that when something appears to be blocking my path in some way, there is an opportunity close by. Success in any sphere of life requires a positive mindset. Without the intention to transmute a problem into an opportunity, you can't move forward in your life, and every setback saps your life force.

Maybe you notice that you have a habit of seeing things negatively in certain situations. Remember not to beat yourself up. You have every right to be as you are. But if you can see that being a particular way is causing you suffering, then stop for a moment and take a breath. Once you return to your *natural* quality of mind, positivity will resume.

> '*Whether you think you can, or think you can't, you're right.*'
> Henry Ford

At the age of 15, Malala Yousafzai was shot in the head and neck, in an assassination attempt by a Taliban gunman in Pakistan. The next year

Malala, the youngest ever Nobel Prize laureate, appeared on an American chat show to talk about the importance of education in addressing terrorism.

When the 16-year-old schoolgirl was asked how she would respond to the man who tried to kill her, she replied:

> *'At first I thought that I would hit him with a shoe. Then I thought if you hit a Talib with a shoe, there would be no difference between you and the Talib ... You must not treat others with cruelty ... You must fight others through peace and through dialogue and through education.'*²

Malala's courage and positive outlook after such a harrowing experience were not out of character. It was for precisely these qualities that the Taliban had singled her out. They knew that she had been campaigning for women's education since she was 11 or 12. This is an incredible example of great wisdom at a tender age, and a demonstration of how adversity can be used to enormous advantage. She used the opportunity to transmute a possibility for great suffering into one of tremendous global inspiration.

Everything that arises in your life is echoing something about you. This is life's invitation for you to grow and express yourself as your highest possibility, perhaps even impacting upon the world in a beneficial way. With a calm mind, you can see opportunity in all that arises, even in painful, past events which led to suffering.

So, if you sense that your default setting is more inclined towards being closed-hearted, negative, cynical and doubting, simply return to your *natural* quality of mind, and transform this to being open-hearted, positive, trusting and looking for the good.

2. Nurture Honesty and Integrity

You diminish your life force and fuel your imbalances when you lie, steal, cheat or are greedy. What you say and do to others represents a vibration, and that vibration is being transmitted inwardly and outwardly. So lying to or cheating another may well hurt them, but it will also be harming you, probably even more than them.

You cannot cheat life, and you cannot lie to yourself, everything that you have thought, said and done is recorded in the memory bank of your subconscious mind, and has already been transmitted into the universal energy field of life. The Law of Karma[3] is always acting, and whilst it has no axe to grind, and is utterly impartial, it never lies, cheats, steals or is greedy; it simply explains how you're inviting your life according to your vibration.

When you act in a way which is not in integrity with the depth of your being, this creates inner resistance and suffering. So if you remember that your subconscious mind is endlessly transmitting within your being, and out into the world, it serves you to make sure that the vibration which is transmitted matches your deepest truth.

3. *Give More and Expect Less*

Every time that you SOAR, you reset yourself. You come back to your *natural* quality of mind, where you are happy with what you have, and you don't 'need' anything else. From here, you realize that all you truly want is to share your sense of inner peace and wellbeing with others. You want to give; and not merely material things, but you want to give of yourself.

Giving of yourself in this way ensures an endless stream of love returning to you, since the vibration that you put out is what you attract back to yourself. As I said in the introduction:

> *'When you give of yourself willingly, you open yourself to receiving many times in return, and your gratitude for this feeds you deeply. The happier you are, the healthier you are and the greater your life force is.'*

When you are in your *normal* state of mind, your heart is contracted, and you don't really feel like giving. Sure, you might make an effort in some way, but it won't be coming from an open heart. This makes you hungry, because when the door is closed to giving, it's also closed to receiving.

Your hunger creates expectation – 'I should be getting this', 'Why didn't they give me more of that?' The opposite of giving is not taking, but expecting. Expectation arises from a contracted heart, or being in a *normal* state of mind.

Expectations are the 'story' that your mind creates, which it then compares with what is actually arising. Since the expectations are colored by your past conditioning, they are never going to match what actually is, and you therefore feel frustrated, let down or angry. Expectations arise from your databank of memories; they are not real.

Whenever you feel like something is 'missing', or that you badly 'need' something, this is a sure sign of a *normal* state of mind. This quality of your mind is excellent at judging and criticizing. Have you noticed this? Sometimes, it just feels like nothing is as it should be. In this frame of mind, you will be projecting your expectations onto everything around you, and, unfortunately, nothing will satiate this illusory 'need'.

So rather than 'expecting less', it's better to expect nothing at all, in the sense that when you see expectation rearing its head, you refuse to touch it. When you notice thoughts of expectation arising, take a moment to sense your inner stillness – SOAR. What you then choose to think, say or do is fresh, and untainted by memory.

4. *Follow the Middle Path*

Middle path – these two words resolve the majority of human dilemmas, as they urge us to be gentle with ourselves, and steer clear of the extremes of life. It is the disturbed, tension-creating thoughts about what we 'should and shouldn't' do which often reek the greatest havoc with our nervous systems.

So avoid pushing yourself and being extreme, and be particularly attentive to those things that you use as a crutch, or are strongly attached to. Being extreme or obsessive in your behavior upsets your *natural* balance.

Having desires is normal and fine, the problem is when you become attached to superficial ideas, such as 'owning, or being dependent upon, your partner', 'obsessing about your new car', or 'protecting your job'.

None of these 'things' are actually yours, and, perhaps more importantly, none of these are responsible for your peace of mind or fulfillment. All of nature is in a state of flux; it will arise, and then it will fall. Nothing is free from this law of life – human bodies, empires, relationships, houses – all will come into existence, and at some point, according to the mystery of life, will drop away.

**We suffer our desires when we become attached
to superficial ideas about them**

Quoting from Dzigar Kongtrul Rinpoche, *Light Comes Through* –

*'Imagine craving absolutely nothing from the world ... Imagine
the freedoms that come from the ability to enjoy things without
having to acquire them, own them, posses them ... Imagine
feeling completely satisfied and content with your life just as it is
...This is the enjoyment of non-attachment.'*[4]

The middle path of Buddha recognizes that everything is fine in its right measure, so long as it does not involve intentionally causing harm to other living beings. This is a powerful realization, since it requires high awareness to sense when you are veering to the extremes of your habitual patterns. This awareness means that you can also adjust for your particular nature:

If you tend to be lazy, or easily fearful, stretch yourself a little more than you normally would and step out of your comfort zone.

If you feel like this sentence describes you in some way, consider what you could do right now that would take you out of your comfort zone, in a positive way. Would it be something physical, verbal or mental? Challenge yourself not to be stuck in your *normal*, lazy frame of mind. (Write a few words in your journal about this.)

If you tend to be an over-achiever, or obsessive, then slow down and assess what is really important for you to achieve.

If you feel like this sentence describes your general approach to life, take a moment to consider how you could 'slow down' in your life, so that you feel more ease. Select at least one area of your life, or activity, and commit to approaching it differently. (Write a few words in your journal about this.)

If you tend towards an addictive personality, then find healthy ways to decompress and relax, or perhaps seek guidance from a professional.

If you feel like this sentence describes you quite well, consider what new practice or activity you could do to give you greater equanimity so that you are not so obsessive. Select one area of your life, and commit to addressing that differently. (Write a few words in your journal about this.)

Whenever you sense excessive behavior, be more moderate and flow with life, rather than trying to push her. With moderation, you are neither lazy, and nor do you obsess – as I said in the introduction:

*'My invitation is to slow down, relax, and to not be obsessed
with over-achievement and being habitually busy; to nourish
your body without excess or frugality, to feed your mind without
strain or ignorance, and to gently flow with life.'*

With moderation, you tend to live a simpler life, considering deeply what is truly important for you. With this mindset, you no longer pursue the 'superficial "blip" of calm and happiness' that offers no enduring fulfillment.

5. Develop Trust in Life

All of life is inextricably interconnected, as part of a 'Unified Field'.[5] Recognizing that 'all is one' means that you would never intentionally make another being or life form suffer. Since if they suffer, you suffer.

*'Everything is in you. You are not in anything. You can't go
anywhere, because you already are everywhere. The whole
Universe is in you. The Universe is huge, but you are infinite.'*
Satyananda

So when you say that you trust life, what you are really saying is that you trust yourself, at depth. Trusting life is recognizing your essential oneness with the whole of Existence. To know God is to know yourself. To meet the divine is to meet yourself. To trust life is to trust yourself.

By nurturing your ability to listen deeply to your own inner voice of wisdom, you become your own guru. This is a powerful way to live, since if you are able to trust yourself deeply, you stop doubting, worrying, and having thoughts that you need to improve somehow.

Life force is coursing through your body-mind in multifarious forms – your breathing, your thoughts and beliefs, your nervous system, through your blood and lymph, and so on. All the systems of the body, including your detoxification and immune systems, are specifically designed to carry life force in its various forms into, around and out from your body-mind. All of this occurs through indescribably complex reactions which are magically orchestrated by Mother Nature so that balance is maintained.

When you trust life, and therefore the depth of knowing that arises from within you, you are surrendered and in your *natural* state, allowing life to flow just as she needs to. You don't need to concentrate in order to breathe, your brain takes care of this for you. But when you are mentally, physically or emotionally stressed, you become contracted and therefore limit your breath.

So to breathe well, and to maintain great health and happiness, trust that life has it all in hand, and there's no need for you to assist in any way whatsoever, other than to stay calm and relaxed.

In particular, trust that you are manifesting just as you need to, and that you have every right to make mistakes, fail, and be less than you 'think you ought to be'. To trust is to accept that all is perfect as it is, even when it's not as you planned, or would wish it to be.

6. Nurture Flexibility

You will probably have noticed that life rarely goes to plan, hence the saying – 'If you want to make the Gods laugh, tell them your plans.'

If you can accept what arises, even when it's not as you planned, or would wish it to be, then your surrender means that you feel no tension. The ability to adapt, adjust and accommodate for life's ways is a powerful quality.

The previous realization, trust, helps greatly with this. If your trust in life is strong, then you will know that whatever is arising is just as it needs to be. You won't resist it. Instead, you will seek the path of least resistance through adapting, adjusting and accommodating.

Think of a river, and how, if viewed from above, its path is often far from straight. It meanders left and right, endlessly criss-crossing the median line of its route. It does this according to the relative hardness of the rock formations in its path.

There is no 'right way' for you to tread the pathway of your life, but there's definitely an easier route with less resistance, and a harder route full of struggle, where you are resisting what lies in your path. Be smart and choose the easier route, realizing that this is more about your quality of mind, rather than the actual steps that you take.

Choose the path of least resistance

7. Have Gratitude

Having gratitude for the way that your life unravels means that you are sending a clear message into the Universe that, 'I love my life, and I am asking, please, for more things to be grateful for.' Gratitude is the natural outflowing of an open heart, so however it is that your heart becomes touched, you cannot help but feel the upwelling of gratitude.

Many religions and spiritual practices encourage you to consider all the things that have arisen in the day for which you can be grateful. This invites you to be in a positive frame of mind and focus on the good in your life. As Martin Seligman said in his book *Flourish*, gratitude is the most powerful emotion for generating happiness.

As we will discover in the next part of the book, quality of mind is king in terms of your health and happiness, therefore if you regularly feel and express gratitude you will see benefits in all areas of your wellbeing. Life manifests around you according to your vibration, so if you nurture your *natural* tendency for gratitude, your vibration will be attracting outcomes to be grateful for.

Gratitude is an expression of your deep love for life

8. Laugh Easily

By this I mean not only that you allow yourself to laugh freely, but also that you don't take life too seriously. The great Indian Master Osho once said, 'I don't take anything seriously apart from humour.' We humans frequently take life far too seriously, with our mental dramas and the tension that they create in our bodies.

When you laugh, a cocktail of natural health-promoting chemicals (including the magical love-hormone, oxytocin) are released into your system, causing you to feel happy and at ease.

Laughter contributes to the health of your immune system and relieves pain and stress. What seems to be accepted by scientists is that laughter gently activates the sympathetic nervous system, then quickly calms it through triggering the parasympathetic nervous system. Laughter also activates the right hemisphere of the brain, which unleashes your creativity and makes you more sociable.

So laughter enhances your intake of oxygen-rich air, stimulates your heart, lungs and muscles, and increases the endorphins that are released by your brain. It then also relaxes you through slowing and deepening your breath, reducing your blood pressure, releasing your muscle tension, and generally promoting your 'rest-and-digest' response. It is rather like a mild form of exercise, followed by deep relaxation.

> *'You don't stop laughing because you grow old. You grow old because you stop laughing.'* Michael Pritchard

9. Be Patient

Patience is not a quality that runs in my family. My friends often laugh at me because of my unwillingness to queue, or to have patience with the little things in life. And yet, I have spent ten years creating and running a business in India, and I am now repeating the same process in Brazil. For all the beauty and qualities of these two incredible countries, they are not renowned for their efficiency. To say the least, they can be frustrating places, particularly when it comes to matters of bureaucracy.

So how is it that I, who come from a long line of willful, and not so patient, personality types, have been able to find patience with some of the more significant aspects of my life?

As a wise person once said, the answer to a question is usually contained within the question. It's the little things in life that most frustrate me, not 'the more significant aspects of my life'. When it comes to the big things, which wield far more influence over the flow of my life, I am somehow able to take these in my stride.

It's about the idea of control. When I think that I can control something, I am easily impatient and frustrated when things don't go the way that I want. In other words, I easily slip into a *normal* state of mind. But, when it's clear that something is entirely out of my control, I can generally keep my lake monster calm and not react emotionally.

The key is to notice what makes you impatient, and use this as your prompt to Wake Up.

Is it easy?

No. Not for me at least. But what I have realized is that I am very attached to some of my habits. Although becoming frustrated or angry because of my impatience carries with it an unpleasant feeling of tension, there is also something strangely seductive about it – the righteousness of reacting in a predictable manner has a 'comfort' to it. My story about how things 'ought to be' seduces my attention.

This is like having one foot on the accelerator (righteousness – *normal* state of mind) and the other on the brake (desire to avoid tension – *natural* quality of mind).

Being patient, therefore, requires that you, and I, clarify this paradox. You simply need to desire peace of mind, more than you desire being 'right'. Standing in defiance of life, with an inner commentary of 'It shouldn't be this way', is an incredible waste of energy.

Notice what tends to make you impatient, and use this as a trigger for your own awakening. The bigger your issue with impatience, the more the trigger for awakening! Life is always, and only, prompting you to find the path of least resistance. As I said earlier:

> *'If you behave as though whatever arises is precisely what you have asked for, then you will magically transform your life.'*

10. Love

In so many ways, this one word says it all. Love is as vital as the blood in our veins. Without it, we perish, slowly, from within. When it is plentiful, we thrive and we 'come alive'.

Opening yourself to giving and receiving love is, in my view, the essential purpose for us humans. It creates harmony, and ensures co-operation and trust rather than competition and distrust. A lovely way of opening yourself to more love is to ask yourself this question –

'If I had more love flowing through me right now, what would I think, say or do differently?'

Even though it's said, 'To err is human, to forgive divine', when there's an abundance of love flowing through you, there is never a need to forgive. If you're able to catch yourself in your moments of judging yourself and others, and therefore you don't cut off the flow of love, then there won't be the need to forgive. I am obviously not diminishing the value of forgiveness, merely pointing out an even higher possibility.

Love is life's omnipotent force causing your being to expand upwards and outwards, so that you merge with Existence itself.

In Conclusion

Each of these 10 Mantras evoke surrendered acceptance, and they point towards love, since love is what flows when the mind is calm and the heart is open – your *natural* state.

Notes

1. I have changed her name to protect her privacy.
2. '16-Year-Old Malala Yousafzai Leaves Jon Stewart Speechless With Comment About Pacifism', *Business Insider*, www.businessinsider.com%2Fmalala-yousafzai-left-jon-stewart-speechless-2013-10&usg=AFQjCNFL5hSUO9bSn gkZBmno2rYoU9wqmQ&sig2=cSeAp4Atll46zJCHAssZjw
3. We will explore the Law of Karma fully in the next part of the book. The basic premise is: 'As you sow, so you reap', or for every action there is a corresponding reaction. In science this is termed 'cause and effect'.
4. 'Quotes by Dzigar Kongtrul Rinpoche', Likesuccess, http://likesuccess.com/author/dzigar-kongtrul-rinpoche.
5. The basic premise of the 'Unified Field' is that everything is held within an interconnected vibrating field of energy. I shall talk about this in the next chapter.

Summary Chapter 3

The Power Of Acceptance

It's About Surrender

Surrender is about accepting life just as it is – whatever you are experiencing in your mind, emotions and body. This means allowing thoughts to float by which you don't want to engage with, without resisting them; and if you have engaged with a thought that you have not 'chosen' to have, you can simply drop it at will.

'In the moment you realize that you are in some way resisting life by attaching to an unsolicited thought, a disturbing emotion, or a bodily sensation, and you choose to not continue that thought, or to not give attention to that emotion or sensation, you set yourself free.'

With surrendered acceptance, your expanded consciousness puts you in touch with universal wisdom. When you SOAR, you calm your mind and therefore have the wisdom to determine what you can do about a situation. Whether you can or cannot affect the situation, either way you stay centered and inwardly at peace.

Accept Yourself

I used the example of my dialogue with Satyananda to express that you are *ok just as you are*; and that in realizing this, you calm your mind, letting go of the story about what you 'should' or 'shouldn't' be doing. The key, always, is that you first come home to your *natural* quality of mind, since only from here can you see things clearly.

From here, you realize that:

Nothing needs to change. Nothing is wrong.
I am perfect as I am.

Learning From Life

You don't have to try to grow. All you need do is be aware of what causes your suffering, and then learn to accept it. Growth is like a re-calibration, or a shift in perspective, which life takes care of.

So the way that you learn from life is through accepting everything as though you had asked for it. This way, nothing has control over you or your emotions.

If you can find peace with what disturbs you, you disempower it by ceasing to give it your attention – you let go of it. Once you've shown that a particular belief, person or situation no longer troubles you, life stops presenting you with that challenge.

If you behave as though whatever arises is precisely what you have asked for, then you will magically transform your life.

The 10 Mantras

These are like mini-meditations. When you remember one of them in a difficult moment, or before you need to do something important, simply repeat the words to yourself, until you feel calm. Sometimes just the recollection of a mantra is enough to calm your mind so that you return to your *natural* quality of mind.

1   Be Positive and Open to Opportunities
2   Nurture Honesty and Integrity
3   Give More and Expect Less
4   Follow the Middle Path
5   Develop Trust in Life
6   Nurture Flexibility
7   Have Gratitude
8   Laugh Easily
9   Be Patient
10 Love

Part 2

The Second Key

Take Charge of Your Wellbeing

'Nurture'

Part 1 was a consideration of the essential challenge that we all face as human beings – being in the *normal* state.

I then offered a tool that allows you to return to your *natural* state at will – Wake Up and SOAR. We then examined more deeply why accepting yourself, just as you are, is the key to transforming your life – wherein I offered some mini-meditations: the 10 Mantras, which also invite your *natural* quality of mind.

Part 2 is about understanding that you are attracting your life towards you, and you must therefore take charge of your own wellbeing. Through creating your Personal Support System – the Second Tool – you have the ability to optimize your own wellbeing when you are well, and calm your mind and support your own healing when you are stressed or sick.

So if Part 1 was about learning to calm your mind and therefore relax, Part 2 is about being self-responsible and learning to nurture yourself.

'THE TWO FISHERMEN'

In the beautiful, but treacherous, tidal backwaters inland from the Bay of Bengal, tidal floods rose and surged over the land without warning, and there was the ever-present threat of attacks from deadly Bengal tigers on the land, and crocodiles in the water. On the brighter side, though, there was also a rare, pink-colored dolphin that inhabited these local waters.

There were two brothers who lived here, Arun and Dilip. They came from a long line of extremely poor fisher-folk, as was generally the case in this magnificent but challenging backwater region. Arun was a happy, contented young man, with two small kids and an easy-going wife. His younger brother, Dilip, on the other hand, was a short-tempered father of three, who drank excessively, and was married to a woman of nervous disposition.

This difference in nature of the two brothers is not so strange, apart from the fact that they had both experienced similar challenges in life, having lost their father to a tiger when they were young boys, and frequently losing their homes to tidal surges and the brutal Indian monsoon. Life was tough in these parts, and yet Arun had realized long ago that happiness was of your own making. Hardship had taught him to appreciate the simple things in life, such as the warmth of the sun, the coolness of the night breeze, and the exchange of love within his family that he so cherished.

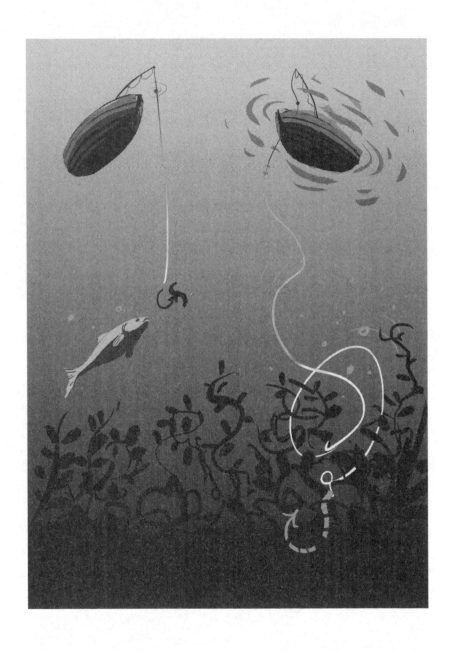

Dilip spent much of the day cursing anything that didn't go the way that he liked. He frequently suffered from heavy migraines, and had gastric problems. Some mornings, the discomfort was so great that he stayed in bed moaning for much of the day.

On these days, Arun would pass by his younger brother's house on his return from fishing, just before lunch, and drop off some of his fresh catch. Dilip's wife would smile timidly and accept the offering gratefully. Dilip pretended not to notice that this was happening.

Arun realized that patience and tolerance were not just of value, but that these were the very necessities of life for simple people like themselves, since life was so utterly unpredictable. You could no more predict the day's catch than the likelihood of the next tidal surge. Unlike most others in the village, he had compassion for his brother, since he knew that Dilip was a troubled man who hid this by living a reclusive life. In fact, Arun himself was an endless source of disturbance for Dilip, who failed to understand why his older brother was always laughing and joking.

Perhaps most of all, Arun was surrendered to the will of Existence, which he trusted with unflinching faith. He recognized that life expectancy for a fisherman was pitifully low in this region, and still he left the house smiling every morning, after kissing his wife and embracing his two small children. Dilip was less surrendered to the majesty of Mother Nature, believing that life was cheating him of what he really deserved – an easy life, with lots of money – and he was therefore harsh with his wife and kids, who rarely saw him smiling.

Arun and his family had many friends, and were very much the hub of the local village. People trusted Arun, and sought his counsel when they had problems, because he always seemed to know what to do. Dilip, on the other hand, felt contempt for many of the villagers, considering them ignorant, and consequently no one ever asked him for his advice, which suited him perfectly since he preferred to be left alone. Arun would sometimes invite Dilip and his family for dinner, but Dilip shunned what he felt to be misplaced gestures of goodwill.

One day, Dilip awoke with strong stabbing pains in his belly and a high fever. The pain was so intense that he asked his wife to fetch the doctor. When the doctor arrived, Dilip was vomiting. His fever grew worse throughout the day. By nightfall he was hallucinating, and by early the next morning he had died.

The funeral was simple and well-attended, as was always the case. What was noticeably different from normal though, was that the only ones who mourned were Dilip's family. Even Arun was without tears, since he, more than anyone, knew that Dilip had never been happy, and was better off free from the shackles of his tormented mind.

Chapter 4

The Law of Karma
You Attract Your Life Towards You

The message of the story is simple –

**Your quality of mind creates your life experience.
So nurture your *natural* quality of mind.**

Dilip chose to be less than positive about life, or at least failed to rise to the challenge of being the best version of himself. His was predominantly a *normal* quality of mind, lacking humility and full of resistance. Arun, on the other hand, had learnt that life flowed much better when he was positive and grateful. His was predominantly a *natural* quality of mind, allowing him to be wise in the face of adversity, and to have a vibration that had a positive impact on others.

Dilip may well have inherited different character traits from those of his brother Arun, but as we will see shortly, modern science is demonstrating that your genes are very much under the influence of your quality of mind and your lifestyle. Whatever internal demons the two brothers had to deal with, one failed to see that he was addicted to his inner story, and therefore 'chose' the path of resistance, whilst the other was humbly surrendered, and sought to nurture himself so that his life flowed. Importantly, we can see that the quality of mind with which they both approached life had consequences for not only their own lives, but also for the lives of others.

The Law of Karma

I mentioned earlier the law of cause and effect, and how this is well expressed through the Law of Karma. According to ancient eastern wisdom, your thoughts, beliefs, words and actions are all causing effects that will come to pass at a future moment in time. (See the illustration of 'The Two Fishermen'.)

In Sanskrit (one of the most ancient languages), karma means action, in the sense that it will generate subsequent effects. So in Indian philosophy the Law of Karma refers to the fact that every action will bear fruit according to its nature – you will reap from life according to what you sow. As is increasingly the case, modern science is pointing backwards to ancient wisdom, and quantum mechanics has proven that everything in life is part of a vast interconnected matrix, or Unified Field. So everything is affecting, and affected by, everything else.

To my knowledge, science has yet to explain precisely how the Law of Karma works in terms of the way in which our thoughts and beliefs attract our lives towards us. That everything is subject to karma is certain, but life promises no certainty about what, when and how things will come to pass – ultimately, it is all a vast, unfathomable mystery. However, Nikola Tesla the brilliant inventor, gave us some insight into this mystery when he said:

> *'If you want to find the secrets of the Universe,*
> *think in terms of energy, frequency and vibration.'*

I see it like this. Thought vibrations within your conscious mind are causing beliefs to be stored as memory vibrations in your subconscious mind. Think of your subconscious mind as a database which records all of your beliefs, and which is much more powerful than your conscious mind. These stored beliefs vibrate with a particular frequency, which then impacts upon your future thoughts, words and actions, as well as being transmitted outwardly into the Unified Field, just as a radio signal is. So the mind is a 'karma factory', and what we believe inwardly is reflected back to us in life. Arun and Dilip exemplified this.

Whilst we may not be able to control what happens to us in life, we are complicit in what we attract towards us, based on what we think, how we feel, and our consequent vibration. Because of this, the Law of Karma is often referred to as the 'Law of Attraction':

You have a vibrating energy field that transmits your beliefs into the world around you, and attracts outcomes of the same energetic vibration back towards you.

Given our capacity for *natural* or *normal* qualities of mind, our thoughts, words and actions are either emanating from a calm, un-programed quality of mind, or they are arising subject to a lake monster which is, to some extent, thrashing about and disrupting the surface waters.

In your *natural* state, you are inviting outcomes which will match your calm and loving vibration, as was the case with Arun. In the *normal* state however, you will be attracting life towards you that will match the vibration of an array of your programed, habitual beliefs, essentially based in fear – as was the case with Dilip.

Once deeply understood, this realization is perhaps the most empowering law of life. Everything in your field of experience has its roots in your thoughts, and your propensity for believing them – the quality of your mind is king. The Law of Attraction therefore describes how your thoughts create your life experience – your 'inner world' is attracting your outer world.

Quality of Mind is King

The Law of Karma also operates on a micro scale within your own being. Your quality of mind is created by your dominant thoughts and most-entrenched beliefs, which affect what you say and do, thus determining your lifestyle choices. Ultimately, therefore, the trajectory of your life begins with your quality of mind, and then follows a karmic chain of events:

'Watch your thoughts – they become beliefs
Watch your beliefs – they become words
Watch your words – they become actions
Watch your actions – they become habits
Watch your habits – they become character
Watch your character – it becomes your destiny'

The origins of this profound quote lie in the Buddha's teachings, and it offers a bird's-eye view of the unfolding of the human experience according to the Law of Karma. It invites us to see why our life experience may often be unfulfilling, if we are predominantly in a *normal* frame of mind.

As you think, so you become

When you are in your *natural* state, you can choose to not give attention to your inner story – your thoughts, beliefs and emotions. From here, you can watch your 'wandering mind and roller-coaster ride of emotions' playing themselves out all day, every day. Like a cinema screen, you can observe the drama of an unraveling story, resplendent with its technicolor imagery – whilst also remembering that what you are watching and listening to is only a story, not reality.

In other words, when you see your thoughts, beliefs and emotions for what they really are – mere vibrations – and you remain detached, you interrupt the karmic chain of events before it gains momentum. You then become the master who sits in observation of your private cinema, enjoying the show, but never mistaking it for reality. This is true freedom.

Don't believe the stories of your mind

Be careful not to misunderstand what I am saying here. I am not saying that you should ignore all of your thoughts and emotions. What I am saying is that when your lake monster is tamed, and with the bright light of awareness, you can clearly choose what to give your attention to. This way you avoid endlessly disappearing down rabbit holes that lead to nowhere.

Please take a moment now to SOAR.

Can you think of a situation where you've observed the story of your mind, and chosen to interrupt that pattern?

Can you see any changes in the outcomes that have manifested in your life because of this?

Whichever frame of mind you're in, momentum is being created. Since so many of us spend much of the day in the clutches of a *normal* state of mind, we will often make less-than-healthy lifestyle choices – how we eat, sleep, rest, work, play and relate to others – which will tend to feed the momentum of a *normal* state of mind. This momentum creates a vicious circle, where a busy, *normal* state of mind leads to poor lifestyle choices which create stress and chronic disease, which in turn invite a *normal* state of mind.

Yet, with a *natural* quality of mind, you will be feeling relaxed and well, and are far more likely to make healthy and supportive lifestyle choices, which nurture your *natural* quality of mind.

Have you ever wondered about the advice to take a few deep breaths before doing something important or challenging, such as speaking in public?

Taking a few deep breaths is a simple version of SOAR. It helps to calm your mind, and therefore allows you to think, speak and act with greater clarity and wisdom, which in turn causes you to feel relaxed and well.

Epigenetics

Whilst still a relatively new science, epigenetics featured on the front cover of *Time* magazine as far back as January 2010. Epigenetics is a new area of scientific study which investigates our genes, and the way in which they influence our lives. 'Epi' means above, so epigentic control means control over our genes. This science is putting forward a compelling argument for the fact that our genes are effectively turned on or off according to our quality of mind, our lifestyle habits and our environment.

According to Nessa Carey, in her book *The Epigenetics Revolution*:

> *'In short, epigenetics is where nature meets nurture. The grounds for excitement stem from the fact that this old and frequently sterile dichotomy is now being fleshed out with real knowledge of how genes are controlled and how they respond to life situations.'*[1]

Who knows what genetic predispositions Arun and Dilip were born with, but what is for sure is that Arun optimized his possibility for health and happiness through taking charge of his quality of mind, making wise lifestyle choices and never behaving like a victim of life. He learnt from life's challenges:

'Arun had realized long ago that happiness was of your own making. Hardship had taught him to appreciate the simple things in life, such as the warmth of the sun, the coolness of the night breeze and the exchange of love within his family that he so cherished.'

Dilip, on the other hand, resigned himself to a life of inner struggle and therefore invited stress and disease. Dilip had only himself to blame for being unhappy, and this certainly won't have helped him in maintaining his health or preventing sickness. I'm not suggesting that his sickness, and his death, were all of his own making. But what is clear is that he refused to accept, or failed to realize, the need to be responsible for his own wellbeing.

Your wellbeing has far more to do with
what you make of your compelling possibility
than how you make do with your genetic blueprint

It was Einstein who said, 'The field is the sole governing agency of the particle.' In simple terms what this means is that invisible forces are responsible for shaping the physical world. Echoing Einstein's words, modern scientific experts such as Bruce Lipton are telling us that 'energy and information fields', not genetics, drive human physiology and biochemistry.

In other words, our thoughts, our attitudes and our perceptions about life (quality of mind) are primary in shaping the way that our genes express themselves. Some scientists are even saying that it is consciousness itself which creates the material world.

This is a wonderful example of how modern science is increasingly pointing backwards to ancient wisdom. Great masters have long said that our mind, once calm and focused, has the power to override our biology, and influence our surroundings. They recognized that we each have a vibrating energy field (aura), principally shaped by the quality of our mind, which impacts upon everything within and around us. So when we think positive or negative thoughts, each has a different impact on our inner, and surrounding, environment. Indeed, 2,500 years ago the Buddha said:

> *'If a man's mind becomes pure,*
> *his surroundings will also become pure.'*

There are many fascinating examples of yogic accomplishments, using psychic powers which are hidden to most of us (*siddhi* in Sanskrit). For example, fasting for tens of days, being buried underground for 30 or 40 minutes without air, and extreme examples of pain management. Since I know one yogi personally who has achieved such mind control, I will offer this as an example.

Clive is a wonderful, lithe yogi in his mid- to late sixties. He has shining green-brown eyes, and a magical elf-like quality to him. Small in stature, but large in aura, Clive told a story to a group of yogis which left a lasting impression. His story was about root-canal treatment – nothing strange about that. What was so memorable about his story were the circumstances, and the matter-of-fact way in which he recounted them.

He told this story during one of his yoga retreats, in Bondla National Park, in Goa, about 12 or 13 years ago. In the middle of one of his afternoon talks, he mentioned that he'd had root-canal treatment. Ever so casually he explained that the dentist was very troubled about the fact he, Clive, had refused a local anesthetic. The dentist had never performed this operation before without anesthetic, and he was reluctant to go ahead, assuming that the pain would simply be too much to bare. I've never had this operation, but I can sense winces of pain from those of you who have.

After quite a discussion, the dentist eventually agreed to go ahead, and sure enough Clive sat there, quite still throughout the operation. No anesthetic, no screaming and no grabbing of the dentist's arm. Clive was able to calm his mind, slow his heart beat and observe the whole experience without becoming emotionally involved. We don't need to replicate the act, but we might be inspired to realize the immense power of our *natural* quality of mind.

Self-Responsibility

With my story about Clive, I'm not suggesting that all traits of character and genetic tendencies can be overridden. What I am saying, however, is that to a great extent, you're not at the mercy of your inherited, or programed, habits and genetic predispositions. You have the capacity to significantly, and positively, influence prevention, healing and the optimization of your wellbeing, through your *natural* quality of mind. This is what I mean by self-responsibility.

I'm certainly not suggesting that you're 100 per cent in control of your own health, since there are far too many potential influences for this to be the case, but you are very definitely in control of your quality of mind – and therefore also your own peace of mind, your lifestyle choices and your happiness. Additionally, in my experience, when you take responsibility for the fact that your quality of mind is the sole determinant of your happiness, you will Wake Up that much more frequently.

You can blame others, poor luck, bad genes and all manner of other beliefs and ideas about your life, but the significance of your role in your own health and happiness is immense, and is determined by the extent to which you take responsibility for your quality of mind and your subsequent lifestyle choices. The difference between the two brothers was that Arun had learnt that life flowed much better when he was positive and grateful – he took responsibility for his life. Dilip, on the other hand, failed to realize his responsibility for the way that he approached life. As a consequence, he did nothing to optimize his own wellbeing, and lived a short, unhappy life which impacted negatively upon others.

Self-responsibility places you in the driving seat of your life. Not to chastise yourself through feeling guilty or worried, nor to pat yourself on the back through pride, but simply so that you feel relaxed and are flowing gently with life. It is my belief that:

**In every moment, with every breath,
you're either inviting health and happiness, or you're
unconsciously opening the door to stress and chronic disease**

For this reason, you must take responsibility for your own health and happiness, through taming your lake monster and nurturing a *natural* quality of mind. As I said in the introduction to this second part of the book:

'... you have the ability to optimize your own wellbeing
when you are well, and calm your mind and support
your own healing when you are stressed or sick.'

The Law of Karma explains how you're attracting your life towards you, and how you have been complicit, to some extent, in all that befalls you. Although you cannot change what you've already thought, said and done, you can release yourself from the apparent grip that these have over you now, through being in your *natural* quality of mind. You are therefore able to create new pathways of possibility, and transform your perspective on wellbeing, sickness and healing.

Please take a moment to consider this. What I am saying is this – your past does not have to equal your future. You current trajectory has no control over your future possibility. The momentum of your current habits may well be strong, but they have no bearing on the truth of who you are deep inside, and therefore the compelling possibility of who you can become – the 100 per cent version of yourself. This is, of course, so long as you commit to taking responsibility for your quality of mind.

Just to be clear, I'm not suggesting that you need to change, or that anything is wrong with you. We've done that one, right? Nothing needs to change, and you are perfect as you are. But, if you feel that something about your life is not working, or you are not feeling fulfilled, then don't look outside for salvation. Realize that you're in a *normal* frame of mind, and all that you need to do is to return to your *natural* quality of mind. From here, you will calmly ascertain what to think, say or do about the situation.

I cannot emphasize enough just how important it is that you keep practicing SOAR. Why? The momentum of your programed mind is immense and takes no lunch or tea breaks. Once it's set in motion it tends to persist. Health and happiness emanate from a calm mind, which is your *natural* state. You know this 'place', and you know how to get there. But if you don't develop your muscle of getting there (SOAR), this 'place' will elude you.

My Perspective

I can sometimes feel like the black sheep of my family. Middle child syndrome, and all that :). I was rebellious from a young age, always wanting to do things my way, and not terribly good at accepting authority. It's probably not so surprising therefore that I ended up becoming passionate about an alternative approach to wellbeing. This opened the doorway to my pursuing, and then becoming, a teacher of yoga, almost 20 years ago.

It's also true to say that in early adulthood, I chopped and changed my passions, which meant that any new ideas I talked about were met with more than a little skepticism. However, health and wellbeing were never off the radar.

I should say, also, that my mother was, by training, a doctor of psychology, and my sister is a renowned professor of obstetric medicine, who married an eminent professor of vascular surgery. One of their daughters is a qualified doctor, and two more are studying medicine at the moment. The fourth is studying psychology. My brother is the head of a language department at an acclaimed UK school, and also possesses a sharp, rational mind!

Perhaps you begin to visualize the picture – me, the yogi entrepreneur, with altogether un-status-quo-like ideas around food, exercise, health and wellbeing – and an entire family of rationally minded academics, of whom 80 per cent are medics. So it is that I have often found myself around a family dining table espousing views that are contrary to the rest of the family. Suffice it to say, there have been a few less-than-harmonious meals over the years.

The fact that I am the 'outsider' in family debates is in part due to my life choices, but it is also significantly down to my tendency to challenge the 'status quo'. I have great respect for my family and their achievements, and science and medicine have made incredible advances over the years. All I would say is that there is a vast realm of ancient, as well as natural, modern wisdom out there, which should not be overlooked. I am, in fact, a big fan of integrative medicine (the combination of modern, western medicine and so-called complementary and alternative practices).

So let me be clear – apart from having studied, practiced and taught yoga for two decades, I have had no medical or scientific training. What I'm going to offer throughout this part of the book is my perspective on health and wellbeing. As I said in the introduction, my perspective is grounded in innumerable conversations with guests and staff at Ashiyana, and 17 years of being on retreats with Satyananda. In places, I shall reference scientific support for what I say, but most of all, I want to appeal to your intuition, and sense of self-responsibility.

Practical Exercise

Please answer the following questions. Before you begin, first SOAR.

- If you think about Arun and Dilip, can you recognize that sometimes you behave more like one brother than the other?
- Are you essentially positive about life, choosing to appreciate the small things, or are you frequently lost in your inner story, and feeling like a victim?
- Overall, how would you say that your life is – is it generally flowing well?
- Can you begin to notice that when it's not flowing so well, it's because of the frame of mind that you're in?
- Can you see that you're responsible for your own wellbeing?

Notes

1. Nessa Carey, *The Epigenetics Revolution: How Modern Biology Is Rewriting Our Understanding of Genetics, Disease, and Inheritance*, Columbia University Press, 2012.

Summary Chapter 4

The Law of Karma
You Attract Your Life Towards You

The Message of the Story:

**Your quality of mind
creates your life experience.
So nurture your *natural* quality of mind**

Dilip's was predominantly a *normal* quality of mind, lacking humility and full of resistance, which caused him and those around him great suffering. Arun's was predominantly a *natural* quality of mind, allowing him to be happy and well, and therefore have a positive impact on others.

Law of Karma

According to ancient eastern wisdom, your thoughts, beliefs, words and actions are all causing effects that will come to pass at a future moment in time – you will reap from life according to what you sow. Because of this, the Law of Karma is often referred to as the 'Law of Attraction':

You have a vibrating energy field that transmits your beliefs into the world around you, and attracts outcomes of the same energetic vibration back towards you

In your *natural* state, you are inviting outcomes which will match your calm and loving vibration, as was the case with Arun. In the *normal* state, however, you will be attracting life towards you that matches your contracted, fear-based vibration, as was the case with Dilip. Your inner world creates your outer world – your thoughts create your life experience.

Quality of Mind is King

Your dominant thoughts and beliefs are creating your life experience, according to a karmic chain of events:

'Watch your thoughts – they become beliefs
Watch your beliefs – they become words
Watch your words – they become actions
Watch your actions – they become habits
Watch your habits – they become character
Watch your character – it becomes your destiny'

Through accessing your *natural* quality of mind, you are able to interrupt this karmic chain of events, and observe your inner world of thoughts and emotions dispassionately. This is important, since your state of mind has momentum, and interrupting your unsolicited thoughts will invite more frequent awakening.

Epigenetics is proving that your genes are turned on or off according to your quality of mind, your lifestyle habits and your environment.

> **Your wellbeing has far more to do with**
> **what you make of your compelling possibility**
> **than how you make do with your genetic blueprint**

Self-Responsibility

Self-responsibility places you in the driving seat of your life, enabling you to feel relaxed and flowing gently with life. It is my ardent belief that:

> **In every moment, with every breath,**
> **you're either inviting health and happiness,**
> **or unconsciously opening the door to stress and chronic disease**

You must therefore take responsibility for your own health and happiness, through taming your lake monster and nurturing a *natural* quality of mind:

'... you have the ability to optimize your own wellbeing when you are well, and calm your mind and support your own healing when you are stressed or sick.'

Your past does not have to look like your future. Whilst your habits may well be strong, they have no bearing on who you are deep inside, and therefore the compelling possibility of who you can become – the 100 per cent version of yourself.

Wake Up and SOAR!

Chapter 5

Taking Responsibility for Your Health and Happiness

All the different elements of wellbeing – health, happiness, prevention, stress, sickness, healing and so on – are intimately interwoven. However, for the sake of ease, I'm going to separate wellbeing into two chapters. This chapter will focus on 'Taking responsibility for your health and happiness', and the next chapter will focus on 'Taking responsibility for your sickness and healing'.

I shall begin with a model of wellbeing which embraces what we've considered so far in the book. It's a simple expression of the factors which promote or inhibit your wellbeing, and is not meant to oversimplify what is an indescribably complex subject.

Your quality of mind is the key determinant of your wellbeing, whether you are healthy or sick, since it offers you mastery over your lifestyle choices, your environment and much of your genetic expression. It therefore allows you to optimize your wellbeing when you are well, and calm your mind and support your own healing when you are stressed or sick.

Your thoughts, your attitudes, your beliefs and your inner 'invisible environment' are more primary in shaping your life than anything in the physical world

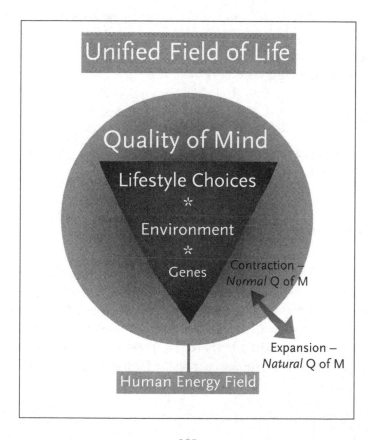

The Unified Field of life represents the whole of Existence. The human energy field represents your whole being (body, emotions, mind, psyche and spirit). The triangle shows the 'hierarchy of influencers' which affect your wellbeing – your lifestyle choices, your environment and your genes.

Normal *Quality of Mind*

When you are lost in your 'story', your quality of mind and your energy field are contracted, and you are prone to stress. Because of this you often make poor lifestyle choices, are more affected by unhealthy environments, and your inhibiting genetic factors are more likely to impact upon your being. If you allow sufficient mental, physical and emotional stress to build up in your system, you will most likely become sick (as was the case with Dilip).

Given the prevalence of stress in our lives today, this has become the primary factor in our fall from health and happiness.

Natural *Quality of Mind*

The more that you are in your *natural* quality of mind, the more expansive is your energy field and the more you merge with the Unified Field of life, and thus the better you feel. From here, you sense your heartfelt desires, and tap into your inner wisdom. You therefore make supportive lifestyle choices, develop nurturing relationships, prevent or support the healing of sickness, and optimize your possibility for feeling happy and fulfilled (as did Arun).

Wouldn't it be better to live with your focus on health and happiness as the *natural* order that you are maintaining, rather than living your life in ignorance and without self-love, and making stress and chronic disease an inevitability which endlessly needs to be cured?

Therefore, your role in your own health and happiness is to live your life in such a way that you are constantly feeding yourself with goodness – like a much-loved garden that has just the right amount of water, nutrients, sun and your own green fingers. Health and happiness (and therefore prevention) are the 'natural order', yet they require awareness and nurturing for their maintenance. In the absence of this self-love you are likely to become sick or emotionally unwell, as part of your body-mind's *natural* cleansing process. As I said in the last chapter –

Your wellbeing has far more to do with what you make of your compelling possibility than how you make do with your genetic blueprint

Holism

The ancient healing arts share a clearly visible thread of commonality, an immutable set of laws defined by Mother Nature, which recognize the interconnectedness of the individual parts that make up the whole entity. The ancient healing systems, therefore, are holistic – they consider the whole human being, realizing that we are more than merely the sum of our parts.

Ancient sages revealed to us that we exist on various planes, or levels of our being, which correspond with the five elements of nature:

- The physical body – earth
- The emotions – water
- The mind – fire
- The psyche (intuition) – air
- The soul (or spirit) – space

In reality these are not separate parts of us, rather they are aspects of our total being which, like all of nature, are inextricably interwoven, where one leaves tracks in the other. For example, thoughts in our mental body become reflected as feelings and emotions in our emotional body, which, if disturbing to us, will express themselves in our physical body as 'blocks'. At the most subtle level, the health of our soul is reflected in all other levels of our being, including the physical plane. Hence the expression, 'The eyes are the windows to the soul.'

So the ancient healing arts realized that for the mastery of health and happiness, a person was required to be deeply attentive to their whole being (with all of its layers). This means a consideration of all aspects of our lifestyle – thoughts, attitudes, emotions, food, sleep, exercise, our actions and so on. For health and happiness to be optimized, everything has to be considered. It is the overall impact of the component parts of our being which determines our overall wellbeing. Whilst they knew that quality of mind was the ultimate controlling force, ancient sages also recognized that the whole of the human lifestyle affected the total picture of wellbeing.

Accepting this is key to approaching the whole matter of wellbeing, disease and medicine. What the ancient sages knew was that if we don't acknowledge the layers of our being, we will never sense the subtleties, and the profound importance, of what cannot be seen by the human eye. And, as modern science has demonstrated, what we can see of life is a tiny percentage of what is actually there.

Your Personal Support System

In today's frenetic world your lifestyle choices are increasingly important for your wellbeing. They ensure that you keep your body-mind vehicle healthy, which makes it easier for you to be in your *natural* state, and thus keep your soul nurtured. In this chapter, I intend to cover the key areas of human lifestyle, and the ways in which they need to be addressed, in order that you are inviting your *natural* quality of mind.

As I said before, I believe that many of the imbalances within modern society derive from two characteristics of our modern lifestyles, and the impact that these are having on our peace of mind. Firstly, that intimacy and loving community have dramatically diminished; and secondly, the fact that we have become so divorced from Mother Nature.

In short, we have lost touch with the customs and health-giving rituals of tribal village life. By this, I don't just mean ancient indigenous tribes, I mean the way in which we all used to live before the industrial revolution. From these root causes, other issues then arise, such as how we eat, exercise, relax and so on.

My point is not that we need to make a u-turn, but that we learn from the wisdom which our predecessors lived by (as indeed many humans do today). My observation about much of modern life, with all of its stressors, is that we need to have a Personal Support System in place. This can go a long way towards replacing what has been lost in our modern-day lifestyles.

The whole of the human lifestyle is inextricably intertwined, and taking care of the more superficial body matters is a part of the whole picture of health and happiness. As the ancient sages taught, the body is the cauldron of transformation, and raising awareness of the physical aspect of our being helps towards the deeper challenge of realizing peace of mind.

Ancient wellbeing systems recognized that each one of us is unique, according to our differing genetic make-up and conditioning. What is helpful for one person may well not be for another, and will likely change over time in any case. So treat this section as an opportunity to explore and discover what works for you, in the knowledge that your Personal Support System will be different from anyone else's.

The intention is that you design your life in such a way that you are constantly inviting your *natural* quality of mind. This means dropping the tendency to unconsciously follow your unsupportive habits. You may notice that I rarely use the word 'habit' throughout the book. A habit is something which generally arises from your *normal* quality of mind. It stands in the way of spontaneity and flow. If you commit to the practice – Wake Up and SOAR – then life constantly informs you about the best way to look after yourself, whether this be in terms of your relationships, how you eat, your form of exercise, brushing your teeth in the morning, or singing in the shower.

Everything begins with your quality of mind. Your predominant thoughts create the all-powerful beliefs which are stored in your subconscious mind. So your most potent beliefs will influence the lifestyle choices that you make. Therefore SOAR (and the 10 Mantras) underlie your Personal Support System.

If you observe Mother Nature you will see impermanence all around. Everything is in a continual state of flux. This is natural. So as you read through these lifestyle points, remember that it is healthy for the specifics within each point to change and evolve. Your job is to adjust, adapt and accommodate for your changing needs.

You may already have discovered great ways of nourishing yourself, other than those which I have included in this section. If so, then great, since finding your own ways to nurture yourself and invite your *natural* quality of mind is you taking charge of your own wellbeing.

I have created the following list to cover the main aspects of human lifestyle. Please feel free to add to it if you feel something is missing for you:

Your Personal Support System

1   Your Tribe

2   Your Relationships

3   Your Environments

4   Yoga, Meditation and Breathing

5   Sleep, Rest and Relaxation

6 Nutrition and Water

7 Detoxing and Losing Weight

8 Exercise

9 Singing, Dancing and Music

10 Compassionate Touch

11 Spirituality and Faith

12 A Coach

At the end of each lifestyle point, I am going to ask you to complete a practical exercise, in the form of a few questions. I will ask these in the first person singular, since I would like you to actually ask yourself the question. The questions will be of this type:

- What does tribe, or loving community, mean for me?
- Do I have any hobbies that require me being outside and breathing fresh air?
- How do I feel about my love relationships?

Please remember that the point here is neither to chastise, nor be proud of yourself. The purpose of these questions is that they cause you to be introspective, and perhaps highlight some areas of your lifestyle which might need attention or adjustment. I would recommend that you use your journal to write down your answers, as well as to note down important thoughts that might arise.

1. Your Tribe

Before the industrial revolution, most of us lived in small villages or tribes, and family, community and faith were at the center of our lives. When we lived in small villages our lives were certainly not easy, but they were uncomplicated and in harmony with nature, ebbing and flowing like the seasons.

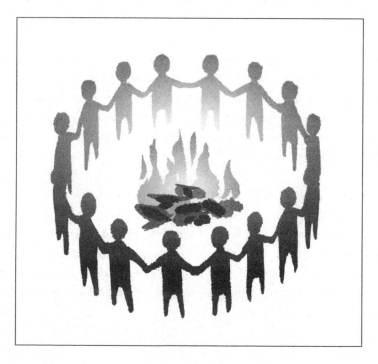

With our modern, western lifestyles, the nuclear family has all but broken down, and we tend to live in vast, sprawling cities. With this tendency to huddle together in burgeoning megalopolises come so many of the heightened social problems that we see today, including stress, chronic disease, crime, excessive consumption and pollution.

The Roseto Effect

Your wellbeing has more to do with your peace of mind than what you eat and how much exercise you do. Life works from the inside out – from the subtle field of the inner body (thoughts, beliefs, attitudes) to the outer physical realm.

For example, if you are totally stressed, then the best organic food will have little benefit. Conversely, if you are relaxed and yet you have a poor diet, then your body will still be able to metabolize what it needs, and rid your system of what it does not. This fact is brilliantly demonstrated by the Italian immigrants of Roseto, whom I first read about in Malcolm Gladwell's book *Outliers*.

In the late 19th century, a group of Italian immigrants crossed the Atlantic and settled in Roseto, Pennsylvania. Until the 1960s or so, these people worked together, ate together, prayed together – in short, they lived their lives in a tight-knit community. They took care of each other, and no one was left to struggle or feel excluded. Interestingly, they had lifestyle habits which many of us would probably not consider to be particularly healthy.

Being Italians, they ate pasta and pizza in large quantities, as well as meatballs fried in lard, they smoked like chimneys, and they drank a lot of wine. Yet, surprisingly, they had half the rate of heart disease, and much lower rates of illness in general, than the national average.

Given the extent to which this community bucked the growing trend of heart disease and other major chronic illness (not to mention the lack of social discord), during the 1950s and 1960s, a number of studies were conducted. One sociologist, John Bruhn, stated:

> 'There was no suicide, no alcoholism, no drug addiction, and very little crime. They didn't have anyone on welfare. Then we looked at peptic ulcers. They didn't have any of those either. These people were dying of old age. That's it.'[1]

Research revealed that these anomalies had nothing to do with the most obvious explanations, such as the water they drank, their medical practices or their DNA. Baffled, researchers ultimately concluded that the reason for their optimal health and wellbeing must have been due to their being part of such a tight, loving community.

As history will attest to, many indigenous tribes were characterized by similar optimal health and social harmony. In spite of certain 'unhealthy' habits, this tribe of Italian immigrants was instinctually embracing the community-based lifestyles of their ancestors, living much as they had done in their native land for millennia.

Happiness and a sense of belonging promote health

This story beautifully demonstrates how social interaction within a 'tribe', and the resulting positive emotional state, is deeply nourishing, and in fact vital for wellbeing. Without this possibility for bonding, humans will not just fall sick, but they will fall prey to all manner of social issues, from addiction, to crime, to suicidal feelings.

Unfortunately, the community of Roseto proved this point doubly. As the youth of Roseto began to mix and settle outside of their tight-knit, harmonious community, it didn't take long before their lifestyles were more like the other people around them. Within a short period of years, the statistics for heart disease, chronic illness and addiction were on a par with the national average.

The Social Problems Of Today

I'd like to repeat the words of the sociologist, John Bruhn:

> *'There was no suicide, no alcoholism, no drug addiction, and very little crime. They didn't have anyone on welfare.'*

The people of Roseto were contented with their lives, and because of this they were healthy and socially well adjusted. This is interesting and important, since it reflects recent research findings that the real cause of addiction and many social problems is loneliness, and a lack of loving community.

When you are feeling lonely and missing some form of community, this creates inner stress – triggering the body's 'fight-or-flight' response.

Research shows that loneliness represents a stronger health risk than smoking or lack of exercise, and may well also cause sociopathic behavior. Hence George Monbiot says in his *Guardian* article, that we are living in 'The age of loneliness'.²

As I said in the first part of the book:

> '*Addiction is so common-place today, as to be the norm rather than the exception. In fact, I would go as far as to say that, to a greater or lesser extent, almost everyone is addicted to something – sugar, food, alcohol, cigarettes, drugs, sex, mobile phones, computers, money and so on. Almost all of us have some "crutch" that we rely on as a part of our daily routine in order to be distracted, to unwind, or to help us deal with difficult times.*'

Most things in moderation will not cause too much harm, but be aware of your dependence upon anything. This does not mean feeling guilty or chastising yourself, it means merely that you be honest with yourself. To accept something as it is, is to bring it out of hiding so that it can be bathed in life's healing ways. It's far better to acknowledge that you 'need' something for the time being, than it is to either ignore it, or to embark upon some extreme mission to cut it out of your life.

This is why I would never advocate that someone give up cigarettes, alcohol or any other deeply rooted habit through extreme measures, since this will cause more harm than good. Extreme measures create tension, and, as we now know, regular activation of our fight-or-flight mechanism is extremely stressful for the body.

If the addiction is serious, you may need professional help. Apart from organizations like 'Alcoholics Anonymous', 'Narcotics Anonymous', other forms of 'The Twelve Steps', and rehabilitation centers, there are also some very powerful and transformative courses and retreats that you can attend around the world.

Recent studies clearly demonstrate that all manner of social problems, from addiction, to depression, to crime and other such unsociable behavior, have their roots in feelings of loneliness and not belonging to some form of loving community.

Loving community provides healthy ways of decompressing, such as dancing, singing and a multitude of other rituals. Human beings are bonding creatures, we need to connect with others and give and receive love. Our modern-day lifestyles frequently deprive us of this 'real' connection, and we satisfy this yearning through artificial, social-media-based connections.

Loving community is key to wellbeing

Practical Exercise

Please answer the following questions. Before you begin, first SOAR.

- What does wellbeing mean for me?
- How do I know if I am healthy and happy?

- Do I have a loving community of people in my life?
- To whom do I go when I am very sad, lonely, anxious or depressed?
- Do I have a shoulder to cry on?
- What does tribe, or loving community, mean for me?
- If there is one thing that I miss in my 'tribe', what would that be?
- What if anything do I think that I am addicted to?
- Does this need or addiction worry me?
- Do I think that I need to seek (professional) help?
- If yes, how might I benefit from this?
- What can I learn from the people of Roseto that I can apply to my own life?

2. Your Relationships

Relationships are the very fabric of life. Therefore, the whole book is really about relationships. Your fundamental relationship is the one that you have with yourself. Not, of course, that there are two of you, but in the sense of how you relate to yourself –

Who do you think you are?

How you behave in one relationship is going to reflect much about all your other relationships. This is because the start point for any relationship is rooted in the fundamental relationship that you have with yourself, and this determines your quality of mind. And as we know, quality of mind is king! So great relationships are determined by your willingness to nurture your *natural* quality of mind.

For most of us, how we relate to ourselves has a lot to do with our early relationship with our parents and other carers – and specifically the way that we absorbed this early conditioning. Many of your mind-made stories and entrenched beliefs that are stored in the vast databank of your subconscious mind were formed in your early years, amidst the joys and challenges of early family life.

There are, of course, innumerable other factors that have affected, and continue to affect, the way that you behave and experience life. Nonetheless, as I'm sure you've already discovered, these formative relationships with your parents, siblings and other prominent early figures, have a miraculous way of repeatedly showing their faces throughout the full gamut of your other relationships.

What is vital to see is that these relationships that you have with your parents and others are ones which *exist in your mind*. As such, they are within your control. You are the master of your mind!

When you resolve the 'stories' of your mind –

> *'I should', 'I shouldn't', 'I'm this, and I should be more of that',*
> *'If only I could have more of this, or more of that', 'I'm not*
> *lovable', 'I'm not good enough', 'I don't deserve this or that',*
> *'pursuing dreams is for others ...'*

And so on, and so on – you pave a solid pathway for all other relationships, including love relationships.

So SOAR, and embrace the gift of acceptance.

Through surrender, you will be able to accept the humanity of your parents and others, and forgive them for what they did, or did not do. This is the key to you accepting your own humanity – realizing that you have the right to be just as you are. Please also remember that there is no time limit regarding your growth and evolution. I sincerely hope that I am still growing and evolving long into old age!

Love Relationships

As is the case with all your important relationships, the 10 Mantras are at the root of a fulfilling and enduring love relationship. I would perhaps just add the words kindness, respect and compassion, which in any case are contained within Love:

1 Be Positive and Open to Opportunities
2 Nurture Honesty and Integrity
3 Give More and Expect Less
4 Follow the Middle Path
5 Develop Trust in Life
6 Nurture Flexibility
7 Have Gratitude
8 Laugh Easily
9 Be Patient
10 Love

Ancient sages thought of these qualities in much the same way as they did a muscle, which needs to be exercised regularly, or it will weaken and eventually atrophy ('use it or lose it'). In some people these muscles are naturally stronger than in others, but they can be developed and made stronger in everyone, through exercise.

Keep practicing Wake Up and SOAR

In the mid-1980s, the Gottman Institute in New York was conducting studies with newlyweds. They called their laboratory the 'Love Lab'.

Their research involved the couples speaking about their relationships, whilst they had electrodes attached to them. These were used to measure their blood flow, their heart rates and how much sweat they were producing.

The researchers analyzed the data and separated the couples into two distinct groups: the 'masters' and the 'disasters'. The 'disasters' looked calm during the interviews, but their physiology, measured by the electrodes, told a different story. Their heart rates were quick, their sweat glands were active, and their blood flow was fast.

Sounds familiar? Our old friend 'fight or flight' at play! The more physiologically active the couples were in the lab, the quicker their relationships deteriorated over time.

The 'masters', however, showed low physiological arousal. They felt calm and connected, which led to warm and affectionate behavior, even when they disagreed. It's not that the masters had superior physiological characteristics to the disasters, but that the masters had created a climate of trust, intimacy and respect that made them more comfortable with each other, and therefore less emotionally and physically reactive.

It's pretty clear to see that 'masters' essentially equates with *natural* quality of mind, and 'disasters' with *normal* state of mind.

Couples who live happily together for years and years look for reasons to connect with one another. They have the awareness to think about the other. A relationship is like a garden, and for it to flourish it requires attentiveness and an abundance of love.

The early relationship that you developed with your parents is pivotal in terms of how you 'see' others. So much so, that if you want to have a great relationship with a love partner, my suggestion is, take the time to resolve your unresolved 'stories' about your parents, with your parents.

Even if one or both parents are no longer alive, there are still many ways to 'have a conversation' with them. If you have trusted friends that you can, and do share with, this may well suffice. Otherwise, I would recommend the support of a professional counselor.

Loving relationships are often considered to be the best opportunity for growth and evolution. This certainly seems to be true. I would like to remind you, though, that growth and evolution have nothing to do with judging and labeling each other, in the belief that they, or you, need to change. Please remember that the start point for everything, always, is Wake Up and SOAR. First calm your mind and relax.

Why?

Because, once you are calm, if you would benefit from being more patient, you will be. If it would help that you listen with more compassion, then you will. If the situation calls for you to get up and walk away so that you calm down, you will sense this and act upon it.

When you Wake Up and SOAR, you place yourself humbly at the feet of Existence, trusting that whatever you then feel to be the right course of action, will be. When you SOAR, you relax and allow your heart to open. When you are open like this, love will naturally flow.

**The essence of any fulfilling relationship is being open to
giving and receiving love –**

So Wake Up and SOAR.

Practical Exercise

Please answer the following questions. Before you begin, first SOAR.

- Who am I?
- How is my relationship with myself?
- How do I feel about my love relationships?
- Does intimacy make me fearful?
- Do I tend to be dependent, or independent?

- Do I look for opportunities to connect?
- Am I generally positive and open to opportunities?
- Am I generally honest and behaving with integrity?
- Do I have the attitude of giving more and expecting less in my relationships?
- Do I generally follow the middle path (moderation)?
- How easy it for me to trust?
- Am I flexible?
- Do I show my gratitude?
- Do I laugh easily?
- Am I patient much of the time?
- Am I a loving, kind and compassionate person?

Please remember that the point here is neither to chastise, nor be proud of yourself. The purpose of these questions (which embrace the 10 Mantras) is that they cause you to be introspective, and perhaps highlight one or two areas which you might like to focus upon. Remember that the key to your wellbeing is a calm mind :).

3. Your Environments

Home and Work

In the same way that our inner environment affects our outer environment, the reverse is also true. We are a vibrating field of energy, so everything and everyone around us is interacting with our energy field, and to some extent affecting us. Other people's emotions will therefore tend to be contagious. In a recent US study of 70 work groups across 51 different companies,[3] it was clearly demonstrated that emotions spread between individuals and across teams. If research was conducted in the homes of a cross-section of any population, we would doubtless find the same results within families, perhaps even more markedly so.

Just over half the population of the world today live and work in vast urban clusters, which are growing at ever greater rates to accommodate the prolific trend towards urbanization. In some of the developing-world cities in countries such as India, South America and Africa, giant slums dot the urban landscape, since vast swathes of these city dwellers are too poor to afford proper housing and sanitation.

In other countries, such as China, there are ultra hi-tech 'mega-cities' springing up to help house the population of over two billion people, who increasingly believe that their future lies in the city. This trend of herding together in giant conurbations, which has been playing itself out for a couple of hundred years or so, is a far cry from the tribal villages of old. As I said in Chapter 1:

'The modern "urban grind" is no longer a pejorative description, but more an accepted trade-off between our "desire for more", and a sacrifice of our health and wellbeing.'

We humans rarely flourish when we live this way, unless we are remarkably resilient to the inevitable stressors. We may well prosper financially, and may also live very active lives, where outwardly much is achieved, but for many of us the price seems to be an ever higher one. I am not suggesting that if you live and work in the city, therefore, that you should move out. What I am suggesting is that you take measures to compensate for this.

Mother Nature

Since many of us spend much of our day in enclosed, air- and temperature-controlled spaces, it's important to spend as much time as you possibly can in the tranquility of unspoiled nature. This has a deeply relaxing effect on your being, and is a wonderful way to de-stress, and regain a balanced perspective. Even if you can't easily access wide-open nature, just find a little space with a few trees, a pond, a small river, canal or reservoir, where you can get a sense of the expansive sky above.

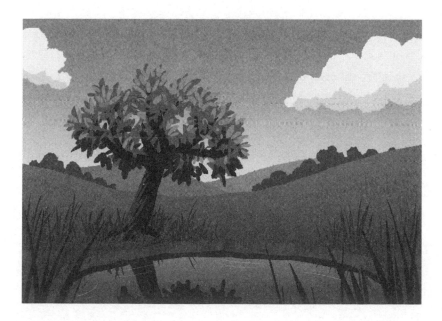

When you do get the chance, get away to the hills, a beach or a waterfall. The air circulating in such locations is said to contain tens of thousands of negative ions, which are believed to produce biochemical reactions that increase levels of the 'mood chemical' serotonin, helping to alleviate depression, relieve stress and boost our energy levels.

It's perhaps interesting to note the following quote about the Lakota Sioux Indians[4] on the matter of nature and the human quality of mind:

> *'The old Lakota was wise. He knew that a man's heart, away from nature, becomes hard; he knew that lack of respect for growing, living things soon led to lack of respect for humans, too. So he kept his children close to nature's softening influence.'*

The Heartbeat of the Earth

In 1954 Professor W.O. Schumann, a German physicist, teamed up with Herbert König, and together they proved that the Earth has a resonant frequency of 7.83 Hertz – the 'Schumann Resonance' – or what we might call the heartbeat of the Earth.

Later research carried out by E. Jacobi at the University of Dusseldorf showed that the absence of Schumann waves creates mental and physical health problems, such as emotional distress and migraines, because our circadian rhythms are disrupted. This effect is likely to be stronger the older the person in question, or the more that their immune system is compromised. When this magical frequency is not present, no new DNA is formed. There is therefore a link between Schumann Resonance and the creation of life.

Today, our atmosphere is so heavily inundated with man-made radiation that it is now much harder to detect this 'pulse'. Considering its importance in terms of our health, this strongly points at the need to get away from the big cities, and into the wilds of nature as often as you possibly can.

Natural By Design

In nature, nothing is straight, or harsh by design. Yet, my observation with a lot of modern architecture, is that rigidity, harsh lines and man-made materials normally override softness of form and nature. Where are the plants, the indoor vegetation, the moving bodies of water, the natural lighting and the natural building materials? Where are the curves, and the flow-lines through a space? Where are the natural smells of nature created by incense, flowers and petals in water, as used in the East?

Be aware of your surroundings and choose them wisely, since we are all, to varying degrees, sensitive to who and what is around us. The more that you bring nature into your life, the easier it will be to relax and deal with stressors.

Sunshine

A lack of sunshine is very depleting for your body, since vitamin D is crucial for your immune system function. There is no substitute for natural sunlight – even just 15 to 20 minutes every few days is sufficient, since Vitamin D is stored in your body. If you live in a region where the sun is less likely to visit, do your best to get away to the sun as often as possible.

Practical Exercise

Please answer the following questions. Before you begin, first SOAR.

- Do I regularly clear the clutter in those places where I spend most time?
- At home, do I have distinct zones – working, eating, socializing, relaxing/meditating, sleeping, stretching/exercising?
- Do I go for a daily walk, jog or bike ride, and breathe fresh air?
- Do I have any hobbies which require my being outside and breathing fresh air?
- Do I make a point of being close to fresh air, water, flowers, plants and trees whenever possible?
- How often do I walk barefoot outside, or lie down in the grass?
- When did I last swim in the sea, a lake or a river?
- When did I last walk in the mountains, or visit a waterfall?
- Do I spend as much time as possible in natural light?
- Am I aware of where the sun is during the day?
- Do I take regular holidays and/or weekends away in the sun and/or pristine nature?
- Do I ever check the sky at night, particularly when it's clear?
- Do I get out into real nature at least once a week?

4. Yoga, Meditation and Breathing

Yoga and Meditation

The essential purpose of ancient practices such as yoga, meditation and tai chi is to still your mind – tame your lake monster. Since, once calm, you become aware of your own inner beauty, which causes you to love yourself and have compassion for others. The more that you are able to attune to your breathing and maintain introspection whilst practicing, the greater the benefit.

To help you in developing peace of mind, you may want to establish a daily practice. Perhaps find out about local classes and groups, or download an on-line class or session. If you're feeling more adventurous, book a yoga retreat or holiday directly, since this may well inspire you to take up the practice more regularly. Personally I believe that one-to-one yoga is the most effective way to learn yoga, and to benefit from the therapeutic possibilities (yoga therapy). There are also many great books and YouTube videos which offer information and guidance about yoga, meditation and all other areas of the healing arts.

In terms of ancient health-giving systems, yoga in particular is proliferating around the globe. This means that for most of us there is likely to be a class which is suitable nearby. Even if you are drawn to a style of yoga or teacher which is not especially oriented towards experiencing inner peace, this is fine, since every path ultimately points in the same direction. It may be that a particular class draws you into yoga, and after a while you find yourself seeking a different class that satisfies a deeper need.

The beauty of practices like yoga is that in their fullest expression they are a complete life-management system, since they consider the whole of the human lifestyle. Yoga encompasses what and how we eat, how we feed our minds, our relationships, how we earn a living, how we exercise, how we relax, how we prevent sickness and heal ourselves, and how we deal with life's challenges.

If you're not particularly open to the idea of yoga then no problem. It's not right for everyone. But perhaps what you can realize is the importance of stretching and moving your body to keep it supple. If you contrast our lifestyles with those of humans just a few decades ago, we are far less active. Our grandparents used to regularly walk, fetch things, kneel down, reach up, and generally keep their bodies far more mobile than we do today.

Posture, Sitting and Movement

'If you don't use it you lose it.' This is one of my favorite lines regarding stretching and bodily movement, and applies to any muscle, joint or line of the body. (In fact, it applies to every aspect of your mental, emotional and physical being.)

My body has always tended to click and crack, and it easily feels stiff. So even though I have a daily practice of yoga exercises in the morning, it is not good for me to stay in any one position for too long. In most instances, this is actually not healthy for anyone. This is why I suggest that you regularly stand up, stretch and change your seat and/or seating position. This is all the more important if your working life involves sitting in front of a computer all day long.

I strongly encourage you to heed this advice. Your body has a natural range of movements. As you grow up, and grow older, this natural range is often lost through laziness, a sedentary lifestyle, or excessive sport and muscle growth. Remember the middle path!

Our posture and sedentary lifestyles have played havoc with the bio-mechanics of our bodies. Neck, back, hip, knee, elbow, wrist and numerous other forms of pain are the norm today. Perhaps the most harmful of our modern habits in this respect is that we sit on chairs, in front of computers, for many hours a day. Many of us need to move more. My morning yoga practice is not that long, or arduous, but I continue to stretch and release tension in my body throughout the day. I would like to be able to do the same postures and have the same range of movements as I currently do, in 30 or 40 years' time.

I am just in the process of designing a new office, within which floor seating will be encouraged. This is to promote sitting cross-legged, or in some way on the floor, and to generally put us back in touch with the floor with more of our body than just the bottoms of our feet. There will be a separate area, integrated within the office space, where you can stretch, lie over a large ball, hang upside down and so on. Our bodies are not designed to be sitting still in one position for prolonged periods of time.

Breathing Awareness

Yoga, meditation and mindfulness cannot be separated from breathing awareness. They all involve the calming of the nervous system, through intentionally (or indirectly) slowing and deepening your breathing. When you are free of any tension – mentally, emotionally and physically – your inhalation begins in your abdomen, lifts up through your chest, and then subsides as your exhalation takes over. At the end of the exhalation, there is a brief pause, before the next inhalation arises.

All the breathing exercises of yoga (pranayama) are designed to enable you to create this effortless, and yet entirely adequate, flow in your breathing – inviting the calming of your mind. When the breath is free of tension, you are home and at peace – *natural* quality of mind.

Anything that you do with your full attention is a form of SOAR, whether it be eating, talking, walking, working or whatever it might be. SOAR, or any other form of meditation, does not require that you sit and close your eyes – this is just one 'form'. So whatever it is that you most love to do, consider making this a part of your daily practice. And as you engage in this activity, become aware of your breathing; this will allow you to 'keep deep roots within'.

For example, if you love to walk amidst nature, in a park or a garden, this can become a walking form of SOAR. Walk slowly, with awareness, sensing your breath as you walk. Maintain a calm, full inhalation and exhalation. As thoughts arise, choose not to give them your attention. This means that you accept them, let go of them in mid-thought, and therefore create no inner resistance to what is arising.

With practice you will realize that you can be aware of the connection between your feet and the ground (this grounding effect is even more powerful with bare feet), whilst still being aware of your breathing.

Staying connected with your breathing is a potent way to invite intro-spection, and SOAR. When you walk or do anything with mindfulness, the beauty around you will be magnified, since it will be perceived through the clear lens of your mind. You don't have to be in pristine nature for this practice to be effective, you can do this on your way to work each morning, or indeed whilst you are doing anything, and you remember to SOAR.

Breath awareness is generally low amongst humans, and most of us are oblivious to the fact that we are often limiting our breath due to a subtle inner tension. As a consequence we are breathing in a shallow manner, high up in the chest. The energy center of the body is just below the navel in the area of the gut (the *hara* in Chinese medicine), so if we are only breathing with the upper part of the lungs, we don't access the energy store of our body.

If you watch a baby breathing, you will see how their belly is totally relaxed, expanding noticeably as they inhale, and then contracting equally as they exhale. They have no concerns about the size of their belly, and if you're wise, you'll share the same disinterest.

With shallow breathing you draw in very little oxygen and life force, and fail to rid your body of stale air. It is therefore very helpful to notice that you sometimes 'forget' to breathe. Maybe you inhale, and due to a subtle inner tension in your gut, you withhold the exhalation. You may also begin to notice how many people habitually breathe through their mouth, or breath heavily while at rest, or perhaps take large breaths prior to talking. Apart from times where there may be sinus trouble, a blocked nose or specific issues, these are all indications of unhealthy breathing.

In yoga, and many other ancient practices, you are encouraged to breath through your nose (unless for a specific exercise). This is because with a steady, easy breath through the nose, you facilitate better oxygenation of your tissues and organs, including your brain. There is a lot of research linking disease with the poor circulation of oxygen!

In addition, the toxins that need to be released throughout the night and day are predominantly released through the breath. As I said before, the in-breath provides what you need, and the out-breath releases all that you don't need, including toxins, tension and tiredness.

Poor breathing is a significant factor in the chronic disease and stress levels of today, since it is both caused by them, and fuels them, creating a vicious circle. If your stress mechanism (fight or flight) has been activated, breath awareness is a potent way to calm yourself down, since relaxed breathing creates a virtuous circle, wherein a full exhalation allows the next inhalation to be deeper and easier. This deep, easy in-breath stimulates the parasympathetic nervous system, which promotes relaxation, therefore helping to alleviate stress and anxiety.

Your breathing is perhaps the single most powerful, transformative tool available to you. It's the link between your inner and outer worlds. The 'quality' of your breathing (the degree to which it is tension-free), is a direct reflection of the quality of your mind. Your breathing is also therefore a direct reflection of your mental, physical or emotional stress levels. Hence the second step of SOAR –

S – Slow down (sit down and close your eyes if possible)

O – Observe inwardly and connect with your breath

A – Accept all that is arising without judgment or resistance

R – Relax deeply and sense your inner peace of being

So when you become aware of your breath, and you connect inwardly, you have the power to directly influence your mental, physical and emotional states. When you consciously breathe more deeply and slowly, you literally create more space within, which naturally invites introspection.

Alone Time

Give yourself ample space to be in solitude and undisturbed by people or technology on a daily basis. You might choose to sit quietly in a room away from all disturbances, or perhaps you take a walk in the wilds of nature. However this 'alone time' expresses itself, let it be a time for SOAR – not doing. This means no electronic devices or games. Through your breathing awareness, connect inwardly and sense how you are. See what you might need in this moment to feel relaxed and well.

Solitude on a daily basis (especially at the beginning of the day) will allow you to nurture your *natural* quality of mind. From here, you will slow your mind down, and easily be able to interrupt thinking about something, or avoid touching thoughts which don't serve you. This will also invite the 10 Mantras to arise as and when they need to:

1   Be Positive and Open to Opportunities
2   Nurture Honesty and Integrity
3   Give More and Expect Less
4   Follow the Middle Path
5   Develop Trust in Life
6   Nurture Flexibility
7   Have Gratitude
8   Laugh Easily
9   Be Patient
10 Love

Alone time includes having space from your lover or partner, in order that you remember who *you* are, independent of them and the relationship that you share.

When you learn to love 'alone time', and therefore also to love yourself, your energy field expands outwards to merge with the Unified Field of life. Anything which then enters your energy field is embraced with the very same depth of love that you have for yourself.

Practical Exercise

Please answer the following questions. Before you begin, first SOAR.

- Am I aware of the incessant chatter (inner dialogue) of my mind?
- Do I know how to calm my mind?
- How does my body feel in general?
- Do I have a daily practice of stretching?
- Can I easily touch my toes? (Please be gentle when you try this)
- Can I crouch down and balance? (Heels off the ground is fine)
- Do I have tightness or a dull ache in any part of my body?
- Do I know where my energy center is?
- During the day, do I intermittently stand up and move my body – perhaps stretching, kneeling down and standing up, sitting cross-legged?
- How is my relationship with my breathing?
- Right now, is my breathing relaxed, full and effortless?
- Can I take several full, deep breaths without difficulty or pain?
- Am I ever aware of my breathing?
- Do I ever take a few full, deep breaths when I notice that I am stressed?
- When I'm exercising am I ever aware of my breathing?
- How do I feel about being on my own? (Ideally you are alone now, as you answer these questions)
- Do I intentionally have alone time at some point of the day?
- Am I ever away from all mobile/smart devices or computers apart from when I'm showering?

5. Sleep, Rest And Relaxation

Sleep, Rest and Relaxation

I use the tool SOAR every night whilst lying in bed. It allows me to fall asleep rapidly, and have eight or nine hours of restful sleep. When my mind is calm the need for sleep takes over, and the slumber which follows is deep and replenishing.

Sleep is, perhaps, the single most potent way to overcome problems and avoid stress. Your capacity for clear, calm thinking is dependent upon the health of your nervous system, and most of all this requires sufficient rest and relaxation. Many of our most difficult moments in life are due to our being tired, emotionally drained and in need of more sleep.

A good night's sleep means sufficient time asleep, as well as restful sleep. Even if your life is predominantly sedentary and outwardly un-pressured, it may well be that your mind is very busy and you are therefore mentally and emotionally tired. Apart from sufficient sleep, regular breaks during the day will also help. The cumulative effect of more restful sleep and plenty of relaxation will be to relax your nervous system, replenish energy, increase productivity, improve attention and memory, and encourage creativity.

Sleep and deep relaxation restore your hormone and cortisol levels (as well as aiding vital body-mind functions such as cellular repair) in order that your body can deal with stress, and be able to heal itself. There is also increasing evidence that dreaming is important for the release of emotional tension and worries.

Around two-thirds of all Bhutanese people get at least eight hours of sleep per night. This is considerably more than the average for industrialized countries. Interestingly, Bhutan is also the country that is famous for the importance placed on happiness – in 1972 King Jigme came up with his ingenious notion of 'gross national happiness'.

Sufficient, restful sleep is key for happiness, calmness, productivity, and overall health

Every human body-mind is unique, and only you will be able to establish how many hours of sleep, rest and relaxation you require. But in order to sense this, you will perhaps need to challenge a few of your habits, such as being overly stimulated before going to bed. A tell-tale sign is when you go on holiday and you spend much of the time sleeping.

Like the wise tribal healers of yesteryear, Dr Naiman, a prominent US psychologist, realized early in his career that it was difficult for people to function well in life, or to address and heal their emotional issues, if they were tired or unrested. His research highlights some valuable points, such as: going to bed early enough; ensuring that your bedroom is dark, quiet, cool and free of electromagnetic fields; relaxing yourself before going to bed so that you are not stimulated; and making a conscious decision to value your sleep and rest time.

Rest and relaxation is an intrinsic part of nature, and a fundamental aspect of 'cleansing and renewal'. Since our sympathetic nervous system ('fight or flight') is so often triggered, it is important that we give our body-mind the time to rest. If we are particularly prone to stress, then slowing down, resting more and sleeping for sufficient time are critical for daily detoxification and rejuvenation, without which we will endlessly suffer from stress and disease.

Sleep problems often result from being worried or overly stimulated, and are a clear sign that you need more rest, relaxation and quiet time. So apart from Dr Naiman's suggestions, switch off the wifi when you go to bed and keep your mobile phone away from your bedside. Detoxing will certainly help here too, as well as other simpler rituals such as using a drop or two of lavender essential oil on your pillow.

If you are stimulating your senses shortly before going to bed, then the mind will be busy. Computers, mobile phones and televisions are all stimulants which affect your quality of mind. Equally, if you eat shortly before going to bed, or you go to bed drunk or under the influence of something, then the body-mind is not ready for restful sleep, as it is metabolizing food or dealing with toxins.

So even if you are exhausted, it is quite possible that you will not sleep soundly. The best preparation for bed is the use of practices designed to calm the mind and invite the relaxation of the body. Taking a warm or hot shower before bed is a wonderful way of cleansing your body-mind of the day. Alternatively, sitting quietly reading a book (which is not stimulating), or meditating is a perfect way to slow the mind. As I said earlier, I SOAR every night before falling asleep.

In Japanese homes, you sometimes see room design intended to create a 'gradual movement towards the bed'. This invites gentle relaxation, so that, as you are about to get into bed, you are already calm and ready to gently drift off.

If you have trouble falling asleep after following the above guidelines, then consult an expert.

Slowing Down

Slowing down is a wonderful way to relax and avoid stressing the nervous system. Hence, it is the first step in SOAR. When you have the awareness, consider talking more slowly, driving more slowly, walking more slowly, eating more slowly, doing your teeth more slowly, dressing more slowly, and so on. In certain situations, you may even find that with increased attentiveness, you sometimes don't want to move or speak at all.

Given the predominant trends of today, where many of us live our lives at high speed with seemingly ever-greater pressures, the primary requirement for most humans is merely to slow down. I recently saw a YouTube video about the 'Slow Movement', a wonderful initiative inviting us to slow down in all that we do. Slowing down activates the parasympathetic nervous system (the brake), and therefore causes us to relax. But it also offers us a reminder to raise our awareness during all of our daily activities.

Slowing down allows us to watch the movie of our life dispassionately, and to not be caught up in habitual patterns. For many of us, the pace of life today is way faster than it really needs to be. Perhaps you can begin to choose the pace at which you want to navigate life, rather than unconsciously subscribing to the status quo of 'speed'. Remember the depleting effects of 'fight or flight', when it is activated regularly and unnecessarily.

When I was in my early thirties, I had a repeating voice in my head telling me that I needed to 'slow down'. It was so prevalent I couldn't ignore it. And over time, I didn't want to ignore it. I recognized that it was life talking calmly and clearly to me. So I stopped what I was doing – chasing recognition and the 'superficial blip of happiness' – and instead I took up yoga and immersed myself in the world of wellbeing. My life took a very different direction, and I've never looked back.

If you visit emerging world regions, where there is little or no impact from the outside world, you will clearly observe that these village people live slow, easy lives that have barely changed in the last few thousand years. Indeed, until enough of them become seduced by promises of greater happiness and pleasure from western excess, consumerism and convenience they have no interest in changing at all. Whilst they may lack modern sanitation, education and opportunities, they enjoy simple lives that are naturally fulfilling, and which are entirely in tune with Mother Nature.

I invite you to see just how powerful it is to slow down for a moment; and perhaps sit down quietly. Take a few deep breaths, and then see what emerges from the depth of your being. When doing this, please remember the third step of SOAR:

Step 3: Accept all that is arising – As you focus on your breathing, let your thoughts flow without engaging with them. Simply choose not to touch them as they arise, and stay more interested in your breathing. If you find yourself momentarily lost in thought, bring your attention back to your breathing (keep doing this until it becomes more effortless).

This is so important, since it reminds you not to be troubled by any incessant, troubling thoughts, or uncomfortable, bodily sensations.

Holidays, Hobbies and Retreats

I have been extremely fortunate in my life to have been able to take regular holidays. These days, however, without wanting to sound like I'm gloating, life sometimes feels like one long holiday. This is probably because I have my own business and spend much of my time doing what I love to do, surrounded by people that I really like. I also have the opportunity to spend much of my time in stunning tropical climes, where nature is both beautiful and abundant.

I rarely feel like I'm working because I love what I do, and since my work is so diverse, it feels like a collection of hobbies. But I do of course recognize that I am perhaps not the norm. So, my suggestion is that you absolutely prioritize holidays and hobbies. And by hobbies, I mean doing what you most love to do, assuming that this is not already your main work activity.

No one can say how often, or in which way, you should indulge your penchant for holidays, hobbies and retreats. The beauty of life is that we are all so wonderfully unique. Because of this, you get to choose exactly how you spend your spare time. I understand that some people are extremely busy at work, or have children to look after, or are perhaps in some way limited by time or money. Whatever the case, remember that your life is yours, and you have the right to design it just as you please.

If time or money are your limitation, work out your priorities and make sure that you are listening to the call of life from within. Become really clear about what is important to you. Develop deep trust in your inner voice of wisdom, for only this can guide you to the life that you deeply desire. If you need to drop something in your life, to make space for something else which serves you better, well then, do that.

If you need to make more money in order to live the way that you truly want to, then seek guidance from within. This may well result in synchronistic meetings with others. In my experience, whatever is right for you, whether you realize it in isolation of others, or it arises through conversations with others, it must always resonate with your inner being. Trust your own inner voice of wisdom above all else.

Or perhaps you don't need to make as much money as you are, and you would rather relax more, then do that. Life is there to provide for your every need. So long, that is, as what you need emanates from the core of your being – life speaking to you. I am going to explore the subject of doing what you love to do, and pursuing your dreams in Part 3 of the book.

Practical Exercise

Please answer the following questions. Before you begin, first SOAR.

- How is my relationship with sleep?
- Do I often wake up feeling very tired?

- What is the ideal number of hours that I require to sleep so that I awaken feeling fully rested?
- How often do I sleep this long?
- Do I rest my mind during the day?
- Do I allow my body to relax completely during the day?
- How are my energy levels generally?
- Am I productive during the day?
- How is my attention level?
- How is my memory?
- Do I feel creative?
- How well do I deal with stress?
- Do I often eat late, shortly before going to bed?
- Do I sometimes go to bed drunk or under the influence of drugs?
- How frequently am I using my phone, computer or watching television just before going to bed?
- Which of my daily tasks could I do more slowly and with awareness?
- Do I ever calmly 'observe' myself during the day, neither troubled by my thoughts nor my bodily sensations?
- Do I take the holidays which I dream of?
- Do I spend my spare time doing what I most love to do?
- Would I like to earn more money; and if so am I truly prepared to do what it would take to achieve this?
- Do I work harder than I want to, and would I like to have more time to do other things that I love?

6. Nutrition and Water

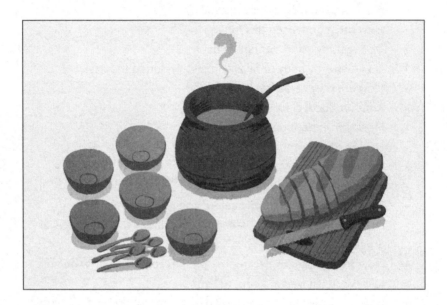

Food and Diet

Ancient tribes instinctively hunted and gathered food that kept them healthy and strong. Everything that they grew was natural, and revered for its life-giving potency. Plants were understood to be connected with universal spirit, and many were known to possess incredible healing powers.

Hippocrates, the Greek father of modern medicine, echoed this when he said:

'Let food be your medicine, and medicine be your food.'

Whilst we live in a very different world from that of Hippocrates, food is still a powerful form of medicine. However, in today's world much of our food is processed and contains additives and preservatives. This is no longer just in the developed world, since the food and drinks multinationals have deeply penetrated the emerging markets also.

On the other side of the coin, many of us have become overly influenced by the swathes of information bombarding us about what is the right diet, and what we should and shouldn't be eating. Given our tendency for stress, we would do well to combine healthy food with a stress-free life. So rather than obsessing about what you eat, aim for a healthy, balanced diet that is delicious, and yet also easily available.

I would suggest the following – whenever possible, buy and consume food and drinks which are closest to their unadulterated, *natural* state. In other words, organic, wholefoods, free range, free of added sugar, unprocessed and not genetically modified (non-GM). Above all else, eat your food in a peaceful environment when you are feeling relaxed. Your digestive system does not function well when you are overly stimulated or stressed.

Also, make sure that you are chewing your food enough – swallowing should be effortless. If you're relaxed when you eat, and you chew your food enough, then you're far less likely to get indigestion, unless you have some specific disorder, or due to medication.

Respect Your Uniqueness

Everyone has different needs, according to their body-mind type, and specific circumstances. For some, raw food can be a wonderful way of increasing vitality and preventing sickness, since it is rich in live enzymes and other health-promoting properties. Yet some people don't digest raw food well, in which case cooked vegetables are a wonderful source of vitamins and minerals.

Since many people also have intolerances, allergies, eating and digestive disorders, and the resulting need for dietary regimes, this area of human lifestyle often requires particular attention, and sometimes the guidance of a health or nutrition expert.

To avoid disease and maintain health and vitality, we need a strong immune system, and food plays a key role in this. For many of us, eating more fresh fruit and vegetables (raw when possible) will give our bodies a blast of nutrient-rich enzymes. Almost everyone would reap the rewards from radically reducing their intake of processed sugar, since this has so many proven negative effects. There are many far healthier alternatives, such as honey, coconut palm sugar and syrup, jaggery (raw sugar-cane), vanilla, dates and so on.

A healthy gut is slightly alkaline. Many people would therefore benefit from reducing the quantity of wheat, dairy, coffee and alcohol in their diet (if they are consuming these excessively), since these products all increase acidity within the gut. Meat is also acid-forming in the gut, but if your body-mind type flourishes on meat, then of course eat it, since depriving yourself will only create stress. Meat eating, and the whole issue of vegetarianism is a hotly debated subject around the planet. I would say just one thing on this subject:

Before you enter into the debate about 'good', 'bad', morality, cruelty and so on ...

First come home – Wake Up and SOAR.

In the midst of a heated debate, no one sees things clearly, so it's better to avoid such conversations until you're first calm. Try to avoid the should's and shouldn't's of life – they always arise from a *normal* state of mind. My feeling is that some body-minds need meat and fish, and others don't. Respect the needs of your body-mind, and realize that you have no idea what someone else might need at this particular moment in their life.

If you're frequently sick, perhaps consider visiting a nutritionist or health expert and establishing a way of eating that works best for you. In my experience this requires patience, trial and error, and above all else, listening to your inner voice of wisdom.

Super-foods

As life always ensures, whenever there is a problem, there is also a solution close at hand. So whilst we live in a world with a proliferation of processed, genetically engineered, and altogether unwholesome foodstuffs, there is also an abundance of delicious, healthy, natural foodstuffs, and even super-foods, readily available.

Super-foods are considered such because of their very unique properties, and when consumed in raw, organic form, they contain far superior profiles of vitamins, enzymes, protein, minerals and many other nutrients than normal food. Consider adding some of these super-foods to your daily diet:

Goji berries, cacao, maca, bee products (honey, bee pollen, royal jelly, propolis), spirulina, blue-green algae, marine phytoplankton, aloe vera, hempseed, coconuts, lemons, avocados, turmeric.

Quoting David Wolfe, the renowned super-food expert:

> *'Super-foods not only help nourish the brain, bones, muscles, skin, hair, nails, heart, lungs, liver, kidneys, reproductive system, pancreas, and immune system ... Consuming super-foods makes it dramatically easier to achieve your ideal weight, diet and food habits.'*[5]

Juicing is all the rage these days, and for many people this is a great way to receive the much-needed vitamins and minerals for a balanced diet. But be aware of just how many juices you drink. Your digestion will always tell you how it feels about your food, juice and water intake. Bowel movements should arise at least once a day. For many of us, it might be two or three times a day.

Without getting too graphic, bowel movements should be fairly easy, and yet the stool should not be too loose. I know for myself that when I overdo the juices, particularly if they contain a mix of several different ingredients, my next visit to the toilet will let me know that the juice was too complex for my digestion.

Hungry?

Hunger can be experienced for a variety of reasons, other than due to the arising of a natural, healthy hunger. For example, hunger can be 'disguised' thirst if you don't drink enough water. In any case, it's important to stay hydrated, particularly if you live in a hot or humid climate. Hydration also requires salt, but try to avoid white table salt as this is highly processed and contains harmful additives, and interferes with nutrient absorption. Wherever possible, use unrefined natural salt (e.g. Himalayan salt, or sea salt).

It's not uncommon to experience hunger due to poor digestion ('leaky-gut' syndrome, for example), wherein insufficient nutrients are being assimilated from your food intake. If you suspect that you might be experiencing symptoms related to this type of chronic issue, then always consult a trusted health expert without delay. In addition, practice preventative health measures by regularly visiting a nutritionist, or other health expert, and perhaps taking appropriate supplementation.

As a general rule it's always better to consume your nutrients through 'real' food, rather than through supplementation. However, if you lack the discipline of maintaining a balanced diet, or the availability of quality, natural foodstuffs, then try to buy high-quality supplements, preferably validated by a reliable source.

Water and Soft Drinks

Again, I am simply offering my suggestions, so please use your own discretion to decide for yourself what feels right.

When possible, drink water that is fresh (from a source), or filtered to remove the harmful chemicals of municipal water (chlorine and sometimes fluoride[6]). How much you require is a very personal matter, and rather than thinking two, three or four litres per day, my suggestion is to listen inwardly and sense your needs.

Here are four reasons to drink more water:

- Dehydration is a major cause of fatigue and weakness – proper hydration helps maintain clear thinking and better concentration
- Consuming enough water hydrates your skin, diminishes the appearance of wrinkles and helps to flush toxins from your body
- Staying hydrated ensures that organs function optimally, which increases your metabolism, allowing you to burn more fat
- Water allows nutrients and oxygen to travel to organs and cells – regulating body temperature and protecting joints and organs

It's estimated that soft drinks kill 180,000 people per year,[7] essentially because of the artificial sweeteners that they use. So if you like canned or bottled drinks, which are full of additives and artificial sweeteners, perhaps consider reducing the quantity that you (and your children) consume.

Practical Exercise

Please answer the following questions. Before you begin, first SOAR.

- How is my relationship with food?
- Is my diet balanced and healthy?
- Do I have a diet/eating regimen?
- Do I eat a lot of processed food and drinks?
- Do I eat a lot of refined sugar, salt and other foodstuffs?
- Do I have intolerances, allergies, eating and digestive disorders?
- How is my immune system (Do I easily and frequently fall sick?)
- Do I generally eat my meals in a calm environment while I am feeling relaxed?
- Do I chew my food enough? (So that swallowing is effortless, and I rarely, if ever, get indigestion)
- Do I experiment with, or regularly eat, super-foods or other nutrient-rich foods?
- How are my bowel movements/digestion (At least once per day is a sign of a healthy gut)
- Do I take supplements, and if so why? (No criticism intended, just be clear why you are – and perhaps consult an expert)
- Do I drink enough water? (If you are not peeing quite a few times during the day, then the likelihood is you are not)
- How is my skin? (Apart from such times as adolescence, the quality of your skin will often reflect poor nutrition and dehydration)

7. Detoxing and Losing Weight

Detoxing

Today's lifestyle patterns – particularly our tendency for stress, addiction to digital devices, poor nutrition and toxic environments – means that our nervous system, our immune system, and indeed all the systems of our body, are working overtime. Whenever you are feeling worn out or emotionally spent, your body-mind is informing you that it needs a break from the current pattern. Ideally, don't wait until symptoms of disease and stress are already raising the alarm.

This is what prevention is all about – avoiding the symptoms of stress, burnout and other poor lifestyle habits before they manifest. Frequent toxic overload, particularly in the city, means that many of us now need to regularly detox ourselves, mentally, physically and emotionally. Sometimes this just requires decompressing through spending a weekend by the seaside or walking in the hills. At other times a deeper detox may be required.

With professional guidance, and a personalized approach, detox and rejuvenation retreats, as well as 'cleanses' and fasting, can be excellent ways of resetting your inner gauge, so that you better intuit what you need and avoid burnout. As I have said before, consider a 'no-technology' day, or week, as part of your personalized support system for prevention and optimal wellbeing. As always, be moderate in your approach.

Losing Weight

Above all else, do your best to stay calm and relaxed about this subject. Being happy and overweight is infinitely preferable to being slimmer and stressed. If you do want to lose weight or it is medically advisable, then giving attention to the other eleven points in this section will serve you well.

There are so many contrasting views on weight loss. Some articles and experts tell you that you must exercise as well as manage your diet, whilst others will tell you emphatically that this is not necessary. It's confusing!

If we are honest with ourselves, most of us lack willpower in certain areas, and if this is your 'weak point', then making great efforts to adhere to a rigid diet and exercise regimen will be tortuous, and likely to end in prolonged bouts of self-criticism and therefore unnecessary stress. Try to remember that the only struggles that you experience in life are within your own mind – my advice, therefore, is to not provoke your lake monster.

Because of this, I have a couple of suggestions:

1. Environment – Instead of focusing on what you 'should and shouldn't do', I would suggest creating an environment around you that naturally supports your goals and intentions. If you make sure that your house, work area, car and so on are all arranged in such a way that you are constantly being invited towards your goals, then you significantly diminish your tendency for lack of willpower:

- If there is no high-sugar-content food in your immediate surroundings, you are far less likely to reach for it
- If you tend to drink a lot of alcohol, then avoid keeping it in the house and going out with friends who encourage you to drink
- If you put your bike next to the front door, you make it far easier for yourself to choose to ride to work instead of taking the car
- Have a small tribe of people around you who know about, and support you in, your goals

2. Fasting – When conducted safely and gently (and with the support of a health expert if the process is more extreme than I am about to suggest), fasting is a supremely powerful form of detox. It can also be incredibly simple:

The time between your last evening meal and your first morning meal is a natural fast. Hence the word breakfast, meaning 'breaking the fast'. This fast allows your digestive system to rest and relax before it has to go to work again. Therefore, if you are able to extend this gap, you extend the beneficial fast.

My recommendation is that you aim to extend the gap to at least 12 hours. That is to say, you eat your last evening meal no later than 8pm, and you don't eat anything in the morning before 8am. If it's not a struggle for you, perhaps eat your last evening meal by 7pm, and eat nothing in the morning till 10 or 11am. The alternative, of course, is to eat breakfast as you normally would, and skip the evening meal, or eat it much earlier. In any case, it's extremely beneficial to leave three hours for digesting your last meal before going to bed. In the words of Dr Mercola, an osteopathic physician who trained in both traditional and natural medicine, the basic science is this:

> *'Your body will use the least amount of calories when sleeping,*
> *so the last thing you need is excess fuel at this time that will*
> *generate excessive free radicals that will damage your tissues,*
> *accelerate aging, and contribute to chronic disease.'*[8]

You will find that after a few days your body-mind adjusts, and it becomes easier, or even effortless, to do this. If time allows, a morning practice of yoga, or other form of conscious movement, will assist you greatly in not eating first thing, since you won't want to eat until afterwards. (Or perhaps just a piece of fruit before you begin will suffice if you are hungry.)

In addition, drink a cup of warm water with fresh lemon squeezed into it (boiling water depletes the vitamin content) at some point before leaving the house. Although lemons are acidic in nature, they become alkaline once in the gut. If you drink lemon water instead of a coffee for example, you aid the natural detox and you help to create an alkaline environment in your gut.

Hot or warm water on its own is also a great 'cleansing' tool. It also diminishes the appetite, and hydrates you in a wonderfully healthy well.

A daily detox such as this will, over time, pay huge dividends. Not just in terms of weight loss, but also for your all-round health and for healing. If you choose to go on a fasting or detox retreat (or other retreat that incorporates these), you will be giving yourself a great gift.

Overeating

Whilst on the subject of fasting, I believe that most of us eat more than we actually need to. Over the last few years I have reduced the amount that I eat, with no lessening of physical activity. I haven't tried to do this. I have simply been more in touch with what my body actually needs.

Forget the implications of weight gain for a minute, and just consider this. Your body and it's nervous system have two principle daily functions — firstly, rest and digest; and secondly, various forms of mental and physical activity. When you are physically active, the rest-and-digest function is diminished or ceases; and when your digestion function is active, you neither rest deeply, and nor are you feeling active.

If you take in more food than your body needs, you place a burden on one of its most vital functions — 'rest and digest'. In other words you will be overworking the whole digestive system. I rarely experience mid-afternoon sleepiness these days (due to overeating), and I have a good level of energy throughout most of the day.

My suggestion is that you slow the speed at which you eat, take time to SOAR, and grow more sensitive to how much food you actually need at any one sitting. The 'slowing down' element of SOAR here is the key to sensing your needs, whether this is food or any other daily need.

I vividly remember sitting down to eat with an Indian sage a few years ago. When it came to dessert time, he hesitated for some time before replying with an answer to whether or not he wanted some ice cream.

When I asked him why he did that, he answered, 'I'm just checking to see if I really want dessert or not.'

It's for precisely this reason that I don't refer to SOAR merely as a tool for meditation – that would limit it unnecessarily in the minds of many people. SOAR is a tool for every situation in life.

Practical Exercise

Please answer the following questions. Before you begin, first SOAR.

- Do I generally feel healthy, in an overall sense?
- Could my body-mind do with more rest than it actually receives?
- Do I, or have I, ever detoxed in any structured, supervised way?
- Do I believe that detoxing in some way might help me?
- Do I perhaps overeat?
- If I am 100 per cent honest, how do I feel about my weight?
- What is my attitude towards dieting?
- Have I tried to lose weight in the past?
- How was my experience?
- Would I value some impartial, professional support with this?
- Do I really care about all this? (I'm happy as I am)

8. Exercise

Many people today are suffering from sedentary western lifestyles, devoid of movement and exercise. The form and amount of exercise required is down to the individual, but exercise per se is extremely beneficial for everyone.

According to recent research at Princeton University, physical activity reorganizes the brain so that its response to stress is reduced, and anxiety is less likely to interfere with normal brain function.[9]

As with diet, there are so many conflicting views about which is the best form of exercise. I would simply appeal to your common sense in recognizing that we are all unique, with different body-mind types, lifestyles and goals. Accordingly, the amount and type of exercise that you require for optimal living is entirely personal. Don't feel shy about seeking the guidance of an expert who can observe and guide you.

In most cases, wellbeing requires only a moderate amount of appropriate exercise. So whether you like high-intensity workouts for a short time, endurance training, yoga classes twice a week, or simply a walk in the park, be true to yourself and how you would like to enjoy maintaining a healthy body-mind. If you tend to be lazy, perhaps engage the support of friends or family to get active with you.

If you are a sports or a fitness fanatic, be mindful of the stress that you might be putting on your body. If you could examine the bodies of professional sportsmen and sportswomen, you would generally find that unless they have 'slowed down' at an appropriate age, or incorporated yoga, stretching or low-impact exercise into their regimes, they are suffering from excessive wear and tear.

Ryan Giggs, the Manchester United and Wales footballer, recently retired from professional football (May 2014), at the age of 40. Giggs is a major proponent of yoga within a fitness regime, and attributes his extraordinarily long playing career, at least in part, to yoga.

Giggs's professional instructor, Sarah Ramsden, has worked with players at Manchester United, Manchester City and various other football clubs, and has noticed a growing acceptance of yoga in professional football:

> '*The change in the game over the last 10 years to being faster, sharper, more athletic and more gymnastic is what has really driven the change in attitudes to yoga. Being supple and having good movement patterns helps speed, power, sharpness of movement, efficiency and recovery, and players can see and feel the difference it makes.*'[10]

Perhaps also try to exercise outside, or take up a sport which requires that you are outside, preferably in the wilds of nature (weather permitting). Not only will you probably enjoy it more, but your whole being will benefit from being amidst the beauty of Mother Nature.

Practical Exercise

Please answer the following questions. Before you begin, first SOAR.

- How is my relationship with exercise?
- Do I do regular exercise?
- If not, why not? (Again, no guilt, just honesty)
- Do I think that it would be good for me to do a little more, or a little less exercise, and why?
- Do I tend to be lazy about exercise and fitness?
- Do I tend to push myself too hard with exercise and fitness?
- Would I like to be physically active and supple well into old age?
- Do I think that I will be physically active and supple well into old age?
- If not, does that concern me?

9. Singing, Dancing and Music

When you are fully absorbed in singing, dancing, and playing or listening to music, you become one with the activity – *natural* quality of mind. This means that you are not busy with thoughts about what you are doing, but you are fully engaged with the activity itself. It's as if you become the singing, the dancing or the music.

Similarly, when you are listening to a singer who is totally absorbed in singing, you 'feel' this in the pit of your stomach, as if you are connected with them (which of course you are), and you again become the singing. This is actually a beautiful exemplification of the fact that 'all is one'.

In tribal tradition, singing, dancing and playing music were central to their way of life, and these activities were prescribed first and foremost as the ways to prevent sadness and alleviate emotional upset. I spend a lot of time in Brazil these days, and what always brings a smile to my face is just how readily these warm, friendly people will break into song or dance.

Unfortunately, this most natural of human expressions is often far less prevalent in the modern world, where we simply don't make time for it. Do yourself a favor, and go dancing, sing with your friends, or go to more musical events. These activities are guaranteed to lift your soul. It's almost impossible to feel sad or anything other than joy when you throw caution and shyness to the wind, close your eyes, and dance or sing as though no one is watching or listening. If you are really shy, try the shower :).

Music Therapy

Music therapy is primarily designed to help patients and clients improve their health, or certain forms of cognitive functioning. For example, there have been extensive studies into the improvement of motor skills, emotional development and social skills, and quality of life in general.

Paul Nordoff was a gifted pianist, composer and Professor of Music, who became so passionate about working with children using music therapy, that he gave up his academic career altogether. He noticed that the children responded very positively to singing, improvization and listening to music. In the case of autistic children, for example, music opened up a whole new line of communication which was unmatched in any other way.

Therapy techniques using singing and dancing have precisely the same capacity to 'touch the soul'.

Practical Exercise

Please answer the following questions. Before you begin, first SOAR.

- How often do I dance?
- How often do I sing?
- How often do I listen to music?
- If I don't do any of the above, would I perhaps like to?
- When did I last go to a live performance of singing, dancing, theatre, opera or other event?
- Do I think that I can sing?
- Do I think that I can dance?
- If I don't already, would I like to play a musical instrument?
- If yes, why don't I?

10. Compassionate Touch

It's common sense that a hug at a stressful time, a handshake after an important meeting, or just cuddling at the end of the day helps you to relax. In other words, compassionate touch invites your *natural* quality of mind.

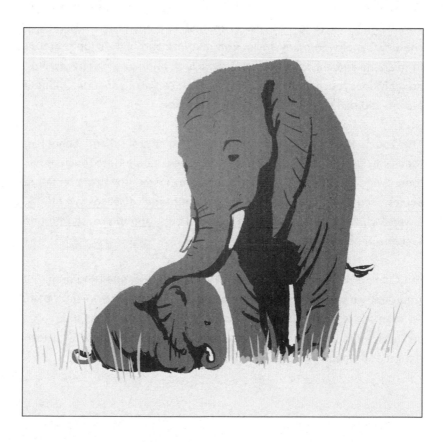

Apart from the physiological benefits, massage, yoga therapy, reiki, acupressure, craniosacral therapy and a myriad of other energy-based healing systems are able to promote a deep sense of wellbeing.

The Healing Power of Touch

Touch was a key component of traditional healing, and fortunately it is now being increasingly studied in mainstream medicine. Research is showing benefits in many areas, from asthma and high blood pressure to migraine and childhood diabetes. Research findings also suggest that not only does touch lower stress levels, but it can also boost the immune system and halt or slow the progress of disease.

The Touch Research Institute, at the University of Miami School of Medicine, says it has carried out more than 100 studies into touch. It has found evidence of significant effects, including faster growth in premature babies, reduced pain, decreased auto-immune disease symptoms, lowered glucose levels in children with diabetes, and improved immune systems in people with cancer.

Jim Coan, a neuroscientist at Virginia University, scanned the brains of (married) women whilst they were being exposed to experimental pain. As soon as the women touched the hands of their husbands, there was an instant drop in activity in the areas of the brain involved with fear, danger and threat. They were calmer and less stressed.

A Sophisticated Tool

Human touch can communicate a number of distinct emotions, such as gratitude, sympathy and love. Touch is therefore a much more sophisticated tool than previously thought. In my view, the healing power of touch is dependent upon the intention and state of mind of the one touching, and the one being touched. Quality of mind is king!

So why is it that touch has such a powerful effect?

Massage, therapeutic touch and any loving interaction cause oxytocin (the bonding or 'love' hormone) to be released into your blood. This lowers blood pressure, decreases the stress-related hormone cortisol, increases pain tolerance, stimulates various types of positive social interaction, and promotes growth and healing. Oxytocin also increases the level of serotonin in the body, which regulates your moods (the 'feel-good' hormone). Not surprisingly, oxytocin is also released through breastfeeding, and even hugging a pet.

In other words, any form of loving, or therapeutic, interaction can activate the parasympathetic nervous system (rest-and-relax response) and aid healing, due to the release of oxytocin. The opposite is also true, and researchers at Ohio State University have proven that psychological stress can slow down the wound healing process.

Is it any wonder that humans (and many animals) love hugging?

Practical Exercise

Please answer the following questions. Before you begin, first SOAR.

- What is my relationship with loving/caring touch?
- Do I like to receive a complementary or congratulatory hug or touch of the arm/shoulder?
- How often do I give or receive hugs?
- Do I like a full-body hug, where I can truly feel that I and the other person are completely relaxed?
- How often do I receive a massage?
- How often do I receive some form of healing or energy-based treatment? (Reiki, craniosacral, acupressure, etc.)
- Would I like to have more loving touch in my life?
- If so, what kind?

11. Spirituality and Faith

Spirituality

At their core, all religions and all spiritual paths have the same intention. They wish to enable you to tame your lake monster, and guide you towards your inner peace of being. They have differing forms – prayer, rituals, practices and so on – but their overarching intention is that you know yourself at depth so that you are untroubled by more superficial, worldly matters. As I said about yoga and meditation, once the mind is calm, you have an abundance of compassion towards others.

I was reminded recently of something that I wrote to a friend, when she asked me a question about how to take care of her daughter's spiritual wellbeing. I replied:

> *'Love her, as you do. That's the beginning, the middle and the end of it.*
>
> *Your love, support and ability to make her feel safe and cared for will give her all the grounding that she needs to make her own informed decisions when the time is right for her to do so.*
>
> *Being relaxed is therefore the greatest gift that you can give to your daughter. The last thing she needs or wants, is you worrying about her future spiritual direction.*
>
> *Chill out – that's the essence of spirituality ;)*
>
> *Chris x'*

The Power of Faith and Prayer

Prayer is meditation in another form. When practiced with deep sincerity, it informs the subconscious mind of what you truly wish for. This is expressed perfectly in the case of my good friend Francisco. In 1979, when he was ten years old, Francisco contracted a rare form of leukemia. His mother was convinced that he could survive this illness, and he began an intensive process of chemotherapy and radiation. Francisco has endured decades of treatment, with many ups and downs, but he has survived. He prays every night, and frequently during the day also. He believes that his ability to stay positive, and indeed the very fact that he is still alive, has much to do with prayer, and his faith in God.

Satsang

Most people have little idea that they exist beyond their body-mind, and because of this they are frequently lost in their story. If you don't have the intention to know yourself deeply, then your experiences will tend to endlessly repeat like a tiresome song.

Satsang is a Sanskrit word which means meeting with Truth. This means being in the presence of someone who is in their *natural* state, and who is therefore also connected with universal wisdom.

I have been attending silent Satsang retreats with Satyananda since 1999, and this has been the greatest influence in any growth that I have enjoyed since then. I am deeply grateful to Satyananda for the tool SOAR. Even though he didn't actually 'give' it to me, it arose, in part, through my contemplating the many conversations that I've had with him.

I would strongly encourage you to explore Satsang, as a way of developing greater peace of mind. There are a number of spiritual teachers, apart from Satyananda, who are offering Satsang and Satsang retreats around the globe, such as Mooji, Eckhart Tolle, Prem Baba, Gangaji, and others. I have included contact details for Satyananda at the back of the book.

Finding the Beloved
'Go directly to that in you which cannot be mentioned
You'll find peace there permanently
It's your diamond, your refuge
It's your self, it's my self, it's the self
Not yours, not mine, it's the beloved.'   Satyananda

Practical Exercise

Please answer the following questions. Before you begin, first SOAR.

- What does the word spirituality mean to me?
- What does the word faith mean to me?
- Do I have a spiritual practice of some sort? (Prayer, meditation, devotion in some form)
- If I don't already have one, would I like some form of practice?
- Does the idea of sitting with a wise person, with whom I can ask pressing questions about life, appeal to me?
- Am I fearful that I would somehow be delegating responsibility to another?

12. A Coach

As I have expressed throughout the book, I believe that life is complex and challenging for all of us. Certainly, over the last 50 years or so, our lives have become far busier, and the demands that we have put on ourselves that much greater. The fact that stress, chronic disease and addiction are spiraling out of control across the planet suggests that we each need to take a good look at ourselves and ask what it is we truly want from our lives. In addition, many people are dealing with recent or past trauma – and whether this has resulted from a car accident, an abusive relationship or the loss of a loved one, the mental, emotional and physical toll that this can take is extremely depleting.

This book is about learning how to relax and take care of your needs on all levels. But as this section of the book demonstrates, there is so much to consider, so many ingredients. It's true that the root of our health and happiness lies in taming our lake monster, and therefore being in our *natural* quality of mind rather than a *normal* state of mind, but this is a considerable, minute-to-minute challenge.

I believe that we all need support and guidance, beyond family and friends, in order to deal with life's travails and optimize our wellbeing. I think that we would all benefit from having a wellbeing coach of one sort or another. I'm intentionally using the word 'coach', so that it's not too specific. In my experience, the person that you choose needs to be the right person for you, and this has nothing to do with the letters after their name, or the 'form' of what they offer. They might be a spiritual teacher, a priest, a psychologist, a psychotherapist or any other form of therapist. The key is how you feel with this person.

I've had various coaches throughout my life. The primary ones have been these: At the age of ten, for one year, I saw a rather conservative, but nonetheless compassionate, psychotherapist; when I was 32, for four and half years, I saw a big, fatherly bear of a man, who was also a psychotherapist; and for the last 17 years I've had Satyananda in my life. Importantly, it was not the techniques which they employed that mattered, it was their love and compassionate listening that facilitated my mental and emotional healing.

Top business people have executive coaches, numerous sportsmen and sportswomen have performance coaches, and yet you and I are expected to navigate this journey called life without any form of professional guidance. Coaching, in any sphere, is increasingly understood to be about 'quality of mind', including in the field of high-performance sports and athletics.

My vision of a coach is not just someone that can help you to 'achieve' though. With today's prevailing trends, I would say that the most valuable aspect of a coach's role would be to assist you in slowing down, relaxing and perhaps having more balance in your life – think 'middle path' from the 10 Mantras. Most people tend to focus on one main role in life, as if this were the center of their lives. Whilst it's great to have a passion, remember the harmonious balance of Mother Nature – everything in its right measure. Perhaps with the guidance of a coach you'll recognize, if you haven't already, that one role of your life strongly predominates, and that you are therefore under-nourishing one or more other areas of your life.

Bronnie Ware, an Australian palliative nurse who wrote a book called *The Top 5 Regrets of the Dying*, said this on the subject:

> *'All of the men (and some of the women) I nursed, deeply regretted spending so much of their lives on the treadmill of a work existence. They missed their children's youth and their partner's companionship ... There were many deep regrets about not giving friendships the time and effort that they deserved.'*[11]

Life balance is not about adding up the hours you spend doing one thing relative to another though. For example, newborn babies, and children in general, may well consume a lot of your daily hours. I'm not suggesting, therefore, that a coach would tell you to spend less time with your kids, and more time out drinking, or playing pool. I often spend many hours writing, or absorbed in one project or another. But if this is what makes me feel vibrantly alive, and so long as I'm not ignoring my commitments, or a deep longing for something else, then no problem.

So life balance is not in the 'form' of what you do, but rather the honoring of your inner wisdom. It's about having integrity with yourself, and trusting that when you are at home, in your *natural* quality of mind, *you* know best. It's my belief, however, that we need wise, impartial guidance to help us to achieve this.

A coach can also help you to consider what is really important for you in your life, such as pursuing your heartfelt desires. When you sense deeply those aspects of your life that truly nurture you, and you give time to them, you take care of yourself on all levels – body, mind and spirit. A coach might also encourage you to take time away from your normal routine, either on holiday, or through spending a few hours in the calm of nature. Apart from the direct benefits, this will give you the space to reflect on how you are, and any ways in which you might perhaps like to modify your lifestyle.

Perhaps most importantly, the coach is not the boss. The coach is there to listen, support and offer feedback. Above all else, they are there to remind you to listen to your inner voice of wisdom – to trust yourself (number 5 of the 10 Mantras). You are in the driving seat; they are your impartial co-pilot, helping you to uncover the road map of your life.

Practical Exercise

Please answer the following questions. Before you begin, first SOAR.

- Do I sometimes feel like I can't cope?
- What does happiness mean to me?
- Am I happy?
- Would I like to optimize my wellbeing?
- What would optimal wellbeing look like for me?
- Do I feel like I could achieve much more than I am?
- Do I sense that I could be happier and more fulfilled if I had a little wise guidance?
- Am I regretting spending so much of my life on the treadmill of a work existence?
- Am I fully enjoying my children's youth?
- Am I fully enjoying my partner's companionship?
- Do I give friendships the time and effort that they deserve?
- Do I have a high-pressure life?
- If so, do I truly want such a high-pressure life?
- Would I perhaps be happier living a simple, laid-back life?
- What is truly important to me in life?
- Do I listen to my inner voice of wisdom?
- Could my priorities do with a little adjustment?
- Would I like to address certain areas of my lifestyle in order to feel happier and healthier?
- Would I like the support of an impartial person in my life with whom I could discuss these questions, discuss my troubles and bounce ideas off?

Notes

1. Quoted in Malcolm Gladwell, *Outliers*.
2. George Monbiot, 'The Age of Loneliness is Killing Us', *Guardian*, www. theguardian.com/commentisfree/2014/oct/14/age-of-loneliness-killing-us.
3. Christina Curtis, 'The one thing standing between you and your success', *Psychology Today* 6 June 2013.
4. '10 Quotes From a Sioux Indian Chief That Will Make You Question Everything About "Modern" Culture', Wisdom Pills, www.wisdompills. com/2015/01/22/10-quotes-sioux-indian-chief-will-make-question-everything-modern-culture.
5. David Wolfe, *Superfoods: The Food and Medicine of the Future*, Blue Snake Books, 2009.
6. The scientific evidence supporting water fluoridation simply isn't conclusive. What is clear is that sodium fluoride (what is actually added to municipal water supplies) is highly poisonous in large doses. (Infants and children are particularly at risk from overexposure).

   A groundbreaking study published in the journal Langmuir11 also questions the benefits of fluoride in toothpaste. 'Toxic Toothpaste Ingredients You Need to Avoid', Mercola.com, http://articles.mercola.com/sites/articles/archive/2015/09/09/toxic-toothpaste-ingredients.aspx.
7. 'Sugary Drinks May Kill 184,000 People Each Year, Says Study', NBC News, www.nbcnews.com/health/diet-fitness/sugary-drinks-may-kill-184-000-people-each-year-says-n384026
8. Dr Mercola, 'Most Americans Eat Too Frequently to Achieve Weight Loss', http://fitness.mercola.com/sites/fitness/archive/2015/10/16/intermittent-fasting-helps-shed-excess-weight.aspx?e_cid=20151016Z1_DNL_art_1&et_cid=DM87995&et_rid=1171635719
9. 'Exercise Reorganizes the Brain to Be More Resilient to Stress', ScienceDaily, www.sciencedaily.com/releases/2013/07/130703160620.htm.
10. 'Yoga Can Help You Stay Forever Young Like Ryan Giggs', *The Telegraph*, www.telegraph.co.uk/men/active/10615428/Yoga-can-help-you-stay-forever-young-like-Ryan-Giggs.html.
11. Bronnie Ware, 'Regrets of the Dying', blog, http://bronnieware.com/regrets-of-the-dying.

Chapter 5

Taking Responsibility For Your Health And Happiness

This chapter focused on your role in your own health and happiness:

**Your thoughts, your attitudes, your beliefs and your inner
'invisible environment', are more primary in shaping
your life than anything in the physical world**

The Wellbeing Model

Your quality of mind is the key determinant of your wellbeing, whether you are healthy or sick, since it offers you mastery over your lifestyle choices, your environment and much of your genetic expression. It therefore allows you to optimize your wellbeing when you are well, and calm your mind and support your own healing when you are stressed or sick.

Your role in your own health and happiness is to live your life in such a way that you are constantly feeding yourself with goodness – like a much-loved garden that has just the right amount of water, nutrients, sun and your own green fingers. Health and happiness (and therefore prevention) are the 'natural order', yet they require awareness and nurturing for their maintenance.

Your Personal Support System

Within this section, I've covered the key areas of human lifestyle, and the ways in which they need to be addressed, in order that you feel well, and are constantly inviting your *natural* quality of mind. This means dropping the tendency to unconsciously follow your unsupportive habits.

Many of the imbalances within modern society derive from two characteristics of our modern lifestyles. Firstly, that intimacy and loving community have dramatically diminished; and secondly, the fact that we have become so divorced from Mother Nature.

Your Personal Support System:

1 Your Tribe
2 Your Relationships
3 Your Environments
4 Yoga, Meditation and Breathing
5 Sleep, Rest and Relaxation
6 Nutrition and Water
7 Detoxing and Losing Weight
8 Exercise
9 Singing, Dancing and Music
10 Compassionate Touch
11 Spirituality and Faith
12 A Coach

Chapter 6

Taking Responsibility for Your Sickness and Healing

The intention with the last chapter was that you design your life in such a way that you are constantly inviting your *natural* quality of mind, and therefore dropping your tendency to (unconsciously) follow your unsupportive habits. With this chapter, I want to explore the role that you play in your own healing.

As before, this chapter expresses my perspective, and I'm going to offer what I believe to be an holistic and integrative approach to sickness and healing. As I said in the introduction to Part 2:

> *'... you have the ability to optimize your own wellbeing when you are well, and calm your mind and support your own healing when you are stressed or sick.'*

Let's begin with a consideration of Dr Mercola's view on this subject:

*'I have long maintained that your emotional state plays a role
in nearly every physical disease ... If your thoughts and emotions
play such a significant role in modifying your biology and your
health (and I believe they do), then treating your emotions
becomes an essential part of optimal health.'*[1]

You will remember what I said about epigenetics, and the way in which our quality of mind, lifestyle habits and environment influence our genes. In the above quote, Dr Mercola is referring specifically to the role that our quality of mind plays in sickness and healing. Accordingly, the Wellbeing Model which I used in the last chapter also applies to when you are chronically stressed or sick. In this instance, your *natural* quality of mind allows you to relax, to make wise decisions about which treatment procedures to follow, and therefore also to support your own healing.

I shall divide this chapter into three sections

1   What is Chronic Disease?
2   Embracing Your Role in Your Own Healing
3   A More Integrated Approach to Medicine

1. What is Chronic Disease?

By chronic disease, I am referring to stress and all other mental, emotional and physical afflictions and diseases which persist for a prolonged period of time. (Some of which you may seek medical help and treatment for and others you may not.)

Ancient healers saw sickness like this: the River Ganges has had many incarnations, principally determined by the state of its cleanliness (or toxicity) according to the amount of rubbish, and human and animal waste that it is carrying. When there is an overload of waste, the river's ability to digest this and maintain its own health is diminished, and it becomes polluted and unhealthy.

Ancient sages realized that our body-mind operates in much the same way as a river – when it is not polluted, it can effectively deal with most unwanted intruders by virtue of our immune system. But when we don't pay attention to what our body and mind are having to digest and deal with, mentally, physically and emotionally, we become imbalanced (overloaded with toxins) and our immune system is compromised. When the imbalance becomes untenable, we become sick.

At the beginning of the last chapter I said:

> *'Your thoughts, your attitudes, your beliefs and your inner*
> *'invisible environment' are more primary in shaping your life*
> *than anything in the physical world.'*

This is the Law of Karma describing how we invite our own sickness and disease. In other words, the determinant of whether or not we become sick is strongly affected by the health of our inner environment – mentally, emotionally and physically:

It is the health of your inner environment (the field) which
determines the effect that outside factors such as germs
and your surroundings will have on your physical being.

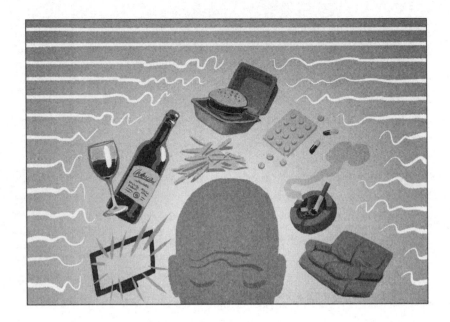

Whilst sickness and health are indescribably complex subjects, we should not ignore our part in preventing sickness, or returning to health if we do fall sick.

Symptoms Are the Language of the Body

Sickness, or any symptoms of less than optimal wellbeing, are not something to be fought, plastered over or resisted – they are sounding a warning as to there being an underlying problem, a clear statement by the body-mind that:

'I need help and support to clean and restore myself as I am out of balance, so please be aware of what you're putting into me, and how you are treating me – thoughts, beliefs, loving community, time in nature, sleep, rest, breath awareness, food, drink and so on – so that I can rebalance myself.'

Therefore, symptoms of sickness and stress, the visible 'hot spots', are not a problem, but a warning of an underlying issue. Stress and disease can be seen as an invitation for heightened awareness, and symptoms may be embraced with gratitude rather than fear.

I have had a couple of chronic issues that were not serious, but were troubling for many years. In both cases, I first tried conventional medicine, and the symptoms simply re-appeared after a few months. It wasn't until I addressed the root causes, through integrative medicine, that the symptoms went away. This meant listening carefully to my body. To facilitate this, I learnt to slow down, quieten my mind and awaken to my intuition. In other words, Wake Up and SOAR.

In this way, my symptoms became my friend – the 'language of my body', rather than some kind of body-mind failure. Everything happens for a reason, this is the Law of Karma. We may well not be able to understand the full complexity of the causes, but we can certainly become more deeply attuned to the way in which our bodies are talking to us.

A good example of this is addiction. It has been considered a fact for some time that many drugs, such as heroin and cocaine, create physical addiction. Yet recent research suggests otherwise. Johann Hari (author of *Chasing The Scream: The First and Last Days of the War on Drugs*) says this about the real cause of addiction:

> '*It is disconnection that drives addiction ... The rise of addiction is a symptom of a deeper sickness in the way we live – constantly directing our gaze towards the next shiny object we should buy, rather than the human beings all around us.*'[2]

Johann uses the example of US soldiers returning from Vietnam addicted to heroin – 20 per cent of them! And yet, magically, 95 per cent of these soldiers dropped their addiction once they re-entered the loving embrace of their families.

In my view, any form of addiction, or deep attachment, is a symptom of a *normal* state of mind. If a person is deprived of loving community, and an adequate support system, they are more likely to be stuck in a *normal* state of mind, and therefore find crutches to lean on. When you deprive a flower or plant of sunshine or water, it wilts, and eventually dies. Humans are no different.

So, as we saw in the last chapter, addiction is a symptom of a deeper issue – loneliness and a lack of loving community. If we only look at the symptom, we focus on the wrong solution. Instead, we need to look deeper at the root cause.

The habitual 'need' for something is an antidote to the normal human emotions caused by social isolation – depression, boredom, loneliness, anxiety, sadness and other such normal states of mind. So, in order to deal with addiction, we need to deal with the root cause – the lack of a supportive tribe and a personal support system. This point was well proven by the people of Roseto!

The Roots of Stress and Chronic Disease

Ancient tribal medicine men and women realized that unhappiness created sickness. They realized the connection between emotions, state of mind and the way in which villagers became sick. They viewed unhappiness and sickness as the soul 'crying', so when a person was unhappy, sick or depressed, it was seen as undernourishment of the human spirit, or a lack of joy and inner peace.

Shaman of days gone by knew intuitively that our spirit is gently but earnestly calling for our attention. It wants nothing material – no jewels, skin-care treatments, Ferraris or iPhones – it wishes only to be observed, recognized and cherished by us. So ancient cultures realized that connecting with the depth of our being, through dance, song, quietness or whatever it might be, was fundamental for wellbeing.

In our modern culture we often have far-less-effective ways of decompressing, such as drinking alcohol, taking drugs or other such activities. These distractions take us further from the depth of our being, causing us to slide towards our default setting of a *normal* state of mind. Not surprisingly, therefore, the view in Ayurveda is that disease begins when we forget our true nature. As I said before:

*'In every moment, with every breath, you're either inviting
health and happiness, or you're unconsciously opening the
door to stress and chronic disease.'*

Your dominant thoughts create your reality. Therefore negative thoughts
bring your immune system down, since the cells in your body react to the
vibration of your mind. Dilip demonstrated this perfectly.

Total Load

'Total load' refers to the sum of all those factors which might impair your
wellbeing. Dr Lipman, one of the leading lights in this new era of holistic
wellbeing, says this about total load:[3]

*'Ultimately, asking the right questions is more important than
giving a label to a set of observations ... This is because most if not
all chronic problems, from heart disease to arthritis, migraines to
irritable bowel syndrome (IBS), depression to fatigue, usually have
multiple factors that need to be addressed.'*

Total load is a beautiful expression of how life's seemingly separate
elements affect one another, and indeed combine to impact upon the
whole. Whether that whole is your body, planet Earth or the Universe,
every single part is intimately connected with every other part. With this
in mind, I have a couple of questions for you:

Why is chronic disease exploding around the world? Why is cancer one of the main killers of humans today, and yet 200 years ago it was far less common?

My view is that a huge number of factors have coalesced to create a level of mental, emotional and physical stress upon our beings (total load) which we can no longer support. Total load means that wellbeing and the occurrence of sickness depend upon the combined effect of all of your lifestyle choices and the environments that you frequent.

It may well be that poor oral health, per se, is not a significant problem for you. But if this is compounded by you being overweight, eating heavily late at night, doing very little exercise, and you live in the middle of a highly polluted city, then the total effect may be greater than your personal 'tipping point'.

Again, please do not start to worry or feel guilty. Even if you have some less than healthy habits, please relax. As we are discovering, the essential key to health and wellbeing is being relaxed and happy – think of Arun, and the people of Roseto. Peace of mind and happiness are a powerful antidote to an otherwise less-than-healthy lifestyle.

I think that it's important to say at this point that even if you, or someone you know, is very sick or disabled, the totality of wellbeing runs far deeper than merely the body-mind. Ramana Maharshi, one of the most famous and influential of all Indian sages, allowed his body to atrophy because he knew that it was merely the outer, superficial aspect of the vastness of who he truly was. Similarly, in spite of being diagnosed with motor neuron disease at the age of 21, Professor Stephen Hawking has become a world-renowned mathematician, theoretical physicist and cosmologist.

True health and happiness lie beyond the body-mind,
since the real you is timeless beyond birth and death

Practical Exercise

Please answer the following questions. Before you begin, first SOAR.

- Have I had, or do I currently suffer from, regular stress or chronic disease?
- Can I see the part that I've played in this issue?
- When I notice the symptoms of stress or chronic disease, how does this make me feel?
- Can I sense that the root cause of these issues lies far deeper than merely the symptoms that are being expressed?
- Can I see that there are perhaps several, or indeed many, combining factors which have led to my stress or chronic disease – maybe my stressful job or home life, plus a lack of sleep, rest, good food and exercise?
- Above all else, am I happy and surrounded by a loving tribe of people, or do I often feel lonely and lacking a loving community?

---

2. Embracing Your Role in Your Own Healing

Epigenetics explains that your quality of mind, together with your lifestyle habits and your environment, can strongly influence your genes. Some experts are even saying that 98 per cent of your genes can be influenced by outside factors.[4]

Your mental and emotional states are key to your healing, because of the way in which they impact upon your subconscious mind and the systems of your body. When you acknowledge this role, you'll understand how important it is that you don't attach to negative thoughts and beliefs about your sickness, and therefore impede your own healing.

As Dr Mercola said,

> *'If your thoughts and emotions play such a significant role in modifying your biology and your health (and I believe they do), then treating your emotions becomes an essential part of optimal health.'*

The Placebo Effect – Your Doctor Within

According to Dr Bruce Lipton (in 'The Living Matrix', www.thelivingmatrix movie.com) science has already recognised that at least one-third of all healing, including drugs, surgery and other allopathic interventions has nothing to do with the process, but has to do with the placebo effect. Dr Rupert Sheldrake, a world-renowned biologist and author, offers the following definition of what the placebo effect actually is:

'The placebo effect refers to the body's self-healing capacity.'[5]

Much like epigenetics, the placebo effect and the whole subject of healing involve deeply complex processes, and the way in which your quality of mind impacts upon your body's *natural* healing capacity is a fascinating and critically important subject worthy of its own library. In my view, the placebo effect itself should be a key topic for funded medical research.

As I understand it, pharmaceutical companies study patients who respond to the placebo effect with the intention of eliminating them from early clinical trials. So it is frequently viewed as a yardstick, rather than the supremely potent healing force that it is. For example, in trials of Tagamet, the anti-ulcer drug that was popular in the 1980s, the placebo was 59 per cent effective in France but the drug itself was 60 per cent effective in Brazil – a difference of 1 per cent. The placebo in one country was as good as the drug in another![6]

I believe that the placebo effect – your *natural* healing capacity, or your Dr Within – is the strongest medicine that we have, for the simple reason that we are a product of our belief systems.

The placebo effect is proof of the fact that Mother Nature has everything under control. Her modus operandi is to always seek harmony, to rebalance what is out of balance, and to heal what is sick. This wonder of nature demonstrates that many ailments can be treated simply by using your mind to heal – the *natural* healing process is enhanced by both your calmness of your mind, and what you believe to be true. For this reason, it's extremely important that you have confidence in the healing system, the healer, and indeed your own part in the process.

The power of your mind is immense ...
The power of your *natural* quality of mind is infinite.

Self-Healing

As I said before, the mind is not separate from the body – hence why I refer to them as body-mind. How you feel mentally and emotionally is intimately woven into your physical being. Having a calm mind, therefore, is the best way to support and catalyze your *natural* healing mechanism.

Healing is principally about engaging the body's *natural* healing capacity, which requires a relaxed and positive frame of mind – your choice about the healing method then supports or hinders that *natural* healing process.

Speaking from my own direct experience, I have been actively involved in healing myself of two chronic health issues. (Neither was serious, but they persisted for many years.) The first time was through using meditation and visualisation whilst working with a homeopath; the second time involved lifestyle choices such as diet and yoga therapy, whilst working with an integrative medical doctor (a doctor who combines modern, western medicine and complementary and alternative practices).

Actively participating in the process of your own healing is not a perfect science, and nor is it easily measurable, especially if you're using several practices simultaneously. But surely it's more important to recognize the importance of your role in the healing process, rather than worrying about exactly how effective it is and why?

When you remember 'total load', you realize that the full process of healing is, in any case, likely to involve various treatments and practices concurrently.

Dr David Hamilton is an expert in the placebo effect, and wrote the book: *How Your Mind Can Heal Your Body*. Here's what he says:

> *'There is no question that the mind impacts the body.*
> *Imagining something, for instance, can even physically impact*
> *brain structure ... I personally believe that we have far more*
> *ability to affect our health and, dare I say, to heal ourselves,*
> *than we have ever thought possible.'*[7]

The Self-Healing Model

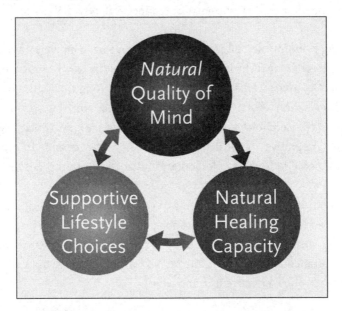

The model opposite (a revised version of that in Chapter 1 showing the relationship between stress, lifestyle and chronic disease) is not meant to oversimplify the complexity of your self-healing capacity. But it adequately demonstrates the need for you to recognize your part in your own healing. Of course we cannot know for sure why Dilip died in the way that he did, but what is for sure is that his unwillingness to take charge of his wellbeing certainly didn't support him in healing his chronic sickness or improving his negative attitude.

I would suggest that your role in your own healing is two-fold:

- *Natural* Quality of Mind – Wake Up and SOAR and the 10 Mantras

- Supportive Lifestyle Choices[8] – Your Personal Support System

Everything begins with your quality of mind. Your predominant thoughts create the all-powerful beliefs which are stored in your subconscious mind. So your most potent beliefs, particularly those about your own health and wellbeing, are the ones that will most influence your capacity for healing. Therefore, being calm and relaxed underlies your capacity for self-healing.

Through your lifestyle choices, you then support or inhibit the healing process. In other words, your Personal Support System becomes your Personal Healing System.

Natural Quality of Mind

SOAR

Step 1: Slow down – If you are not already seated, please sit down now. Check that your back is straight, but without tension. Close your eyes. Take a moment to adjust your position to be as comfortable as possible.

Step 2: Observe inwardly – Focus your attention inwards, becoming aware of your breathing. Make sure that your breathing is slow, rhythmical and effortless. (Try this for at least several seconds.)

Step 3: Accept all that is arising – As you focus on your breathing, let your thoughts flow without engaging with them. Simply choose not to touch them as they arise, and stay more interested in the breathing. Keep bringing your attention back to your breathing.

Step 4: Relax deeply – As you feel yourself becoming more relaxed, begin to sense what is there underneath the breath, before the thoughts. Can you sense an inner ease, a stillness, an expansiveness?

The 10 Mantras

1 Be Positive and Open to Opportunities
2 Nurture Honesty and Integrity
3 Give More and Expect Less
4 Follow the Middle Path
5 Develop Trust in Life
6 Nurture Flexibility

7 Have Gratitude
8 Laugh Easily
9 Be Patient
10 Love

Supportive Lifestyle Choices

Your Personal Healing System

1   Your Tribe
2   Your Relationships
3   Your Environments
4   Yoga, Meditation and Breathing
5   Sleep, Rest and Relaxation
6   Nutrition and Water
7   Detoxing and Losing Weight
8   Exercise
9   Singing, Dancing and Music
10 Compassionate Touch
11 Spirituality and Faith
12 A Coach (including your choice of healer/practitioner/doctor, and the treatment process)

Miracle Cures

The frequent arising of 'miracle cures' (which western medicine is at a loss to explain) has stimulated many investigations into the placebo effect. I see it is this way – given the power of the patient's psyche over their own healing, what they believe, whom they trust, and the treatment processes that they opt for are able to combine and create 'miracle cures'.

Of course there are no rules, and, as always, everything is subject to the mystery of life, but what research reveals is that when a calmly considered, holistic approach is employed (probably involving a number of treatments), the likelihood of recovery is greater, and the recovery more rapid. This is really total load expressed in a positive sense, wherein positive mental, emotional and physical elements are combined to optimize the healing process.

Because of the holistic way in which complementary and alternative therapists and healers often approach sickness and health, their therapies and curative techniques will frequently elicit strong responses within their patient's psyche. Such treatments might include little-known techniques (at least according to mainstream thinking) such as emotional release therapy, meridian tapping, spiritual healing, reiki, pranic healing and herbal remedies, as well as specific, personalized diets. At the very root of all this, though, the patient's peace of mind and positivity is the key.

Dr Wayne Dyer died from a heart attack in Maui, Hawaii, on August 30, 2015, at the age of 75. He was a renowned self-help author, motivational speaker and altogether a rather wonderful human being, who had been diagnosed with leukemia in 2009. But given who he was, and his belief system, he felt sure that he could eliminate this from his body. According to his family, he'd said before his death that he felt that it had left his body. Sure enough, shortly after his passing, Dr Wayne Dyer's family announced that, much to the astonishment of the doctors, the post mortem revealed that there was no trace of cancer in his body.

There are many examples of serious chronic diseases, including cancer, being cured through the use of medicinal plants and specific diets such as vegan, or raw food. For example, in 2003, at the age of 26, Chris Wark was diagnosed with stage 3 colon cancer – usually a (terminal) disease of the elderly. Two weeks later he had surgery and one third of his colon was removed. In a consultation with the oncologist he was told that he had a 60 per cent chance of living five years, and that 'If he didn't undergo chemotherapy he was insane.'

Instead he opted to cure himself through a raw, vegan food diet, plus he embarked upon a rigorous program of self-healing, including naturopathy, numerous alternative therapies such as vitamin C intravenous injections, regular saunas, running, using a rebounder, and he 'prayed like crazy'. At the time of this book going to print, Chris was alive and well.[9]

I mentioned Francisco before, and how in 1979, when he was ten years old he contracted a rare form of leukemia. Whilst his father remained in Brasilia, his mother and grandmother went with Francisco to the United States for treatment. He underwent an intensive process of chemotherapy and radiation, and the following year he had part of his intestine and one kidney removed. As a result of the leukemia he also required a bone marrow transplant.

At the age of 21, because of the damage caused by the chemotherapy, his remaining kidney was failing. However, he was strongly advised against a kidney transplant by his doctor, who said that his body was simply too weak. The doctor also said that he would not survive more than six months, and that he should therefore go home and enjoy these last months with his family. Francisco refused to accept this perspective, and replied, 'You don't have control over me. I am going to find a solution. I am going to law school.' With a kidney supplied by his sister, he had a kidney transplant.

When he graduated from law school, first of 120 students, this same doctor came up to him and spoke with him, thinking that he was Francisco's brother. He assumed that Francisco had died. When Francisco explained that it was indeed him, Francisco, the doctor fell to his knees and said, 'Please forgive me, I wish that I had your faith.'

Since then Francisco has had various, further forms of cancer, including cancer of the tongue, lips and skin. Francisco believes that his miraculous survival is principally due to his faith, his will to survive, and the incredible support and love of his family. Francisco believes that doctors need to be careful with their prognoses, because they really don't know what is possible through the power of faith and spiritual guidance. He believes that we are more than just a body, and through our faith, we can gain immeasurable support from a higher power than ourselves.

Over the years, he has had extensive western medical treatment, but has also taken responsibility for his healing into his own hands. He has a special diet, exercises regularly, keeps his mind extremely active (he's a successful lawyer), and prays regularly. More recently, in part because of my suggestions, Francisco has embarked upon integrative medical treatments, such as ozone therapy.

Francisco is a kind human being, who is humble and full of gratitude. He gives hours of his time to supporting a young children's orphanage, and also visits hospitals and churches to give spiritual support to people facing chronic illness. He surrounds himself with loving community ('Roseto Effect'), has an indomitable spirit, and is a positive human being. His positive quality of mind and his nurturing lifestyle have surely played a key role in his self-healing and overall wellbeing.

I offer these examples not to suggest that all cancer can be cured in these ways, but as examples of what is possible sometimes through the power of faith, belief and love. I invite you to consider that we play a far bigger role in our own healing than we are typically led to believe.

Wouldn't it be better to knowingly participate in your own self-healing, rather than delegate full responsibility to outside forces?

Nurturing your peace of mind, and creating a supportive lifestyle is the essential role that you play in preventing disease and facilitating your own healing process.

> **Practical Exercise**
>
> Please answer the following questions. Before you begin, first SOAR.
>
> - Can I sense that there is a healing force within my being, which will work much more effectively if I 'get out of its way' with my busy mind and less-than-positive beliefs?
> - Have I knowingly participated in my self-healing process?
> - If so, how did this make me feel?
> - How do I feel about 'miracle cures'? Do I view these cynically, or can I see them as part of Mother Nature's indescribably complex and mysterious rebalancing ritual?
> - Do I believe that I can catalyze this mysterious healing power through my own peace of mind and supportive lifestyle choices?

3. A More Integrated Approach To Healing and Medicine

The Dawn of a New Approach

The dawn of a new approach to healing and medicine would seem to be upon us, with the complementary and alternative medical industry (CAM) burgeoning, and a growing awareness that prevention is always a better course of action than relying on cure. We are beginning to see practices such as yoga therapy, acupuncture, herbal medicine, myriad forms of massage and so on entering mainstream medicine.

Indeed the UK Government recently commissioned a report on CAM (www.getwelluk.com), which spoke very favorably of the price advantage, the benefits to the NHS and the overall efficacy of the main CAM practices. I predict that in the not-too-distant future, there will be more than enough evidence for innumerable alternative healing systems to be recognized as valid techniques for the prevention and healing of stress and chronic disease.

So why is a more integrated approach necessary?

The term 'healing' is a very broad one, and necessarily so, since at one level it involves addressing relatively simple imbalances through a program of unwinding and relaxation. At the other end of the spectrum, however, it may well mean a prolonged period of treatment incorporating a carefully personalized program with considerable lifestyle adjustment to heal serious, chronic issues such as cancer or heart disease. Most importantly, though, 'healing' means coming back to an equanimous state of optimal wellbeing, not merely the curing of an apparent problem.

Therefore, to truly effect healing, treatment processes need to embrace an holistic approach which recognizes that the mental and emotional state of the patient is key to the healing process. Ultimately this means a more integrated approach to healing and medicine.

Modern Western Medicine

Western medicine has made some advances which are nothing less than miraculous, particularly in the area of 'acute medicine' – life-threatening disease, complications during pregnancy, transplants, reconstructive surgery, accident treatment, infection, acute pain relief and so on. But there would seem to be some large holes, or areas where this marvelous body of knowledge is less than complete, which the more humble amongst the medical fraternity are openly willing to discuss.

For example, the enduring unwillingness of many within the medical establishment to embrace an holistic approach means that western medicine is generally ineffective in dealing with stress and chronic disease, since it fails to tackle the root cause of the problem. In other words, it seeks to cure the symptoms of the problem rather than actually healing the person.

This issue is compounded by the fact that modern medicine and mainstream science will generally see their traditional 'control tests' as the de facto determinant of what works and what does not. At times though, these tests only serve to support a very limited view of reality. They simply are not designed to embrace all systems of healing, and nor do they take account of all of the elements within the healing process, such as quality of mind.

I believe that in control tests the placebo effect may not be stimulated half as efficaciously as more naturally supportive circumstances might allow. This will be especially true in cases where the patient is intentionally involved in their healing process, as was the case in all three examples that I cited in 'Miracle Cures'.

At other times, tests and statistics are simply misrepresented. In a 'Ted Talks' presentation Ben Goldacre, a crusader for exposing 'bad medicine', highlights the problem with relying on statistics.[10]

> *'All too often in allopathic studies, the full results of a study are rarely published, only those which serve to support what the drug company wishes doctors to believe.'*

Dr Marcia Angell[11] of the Harvard Medical School, and former editor in chief at the *New England Journal of Medicine*, confirms this point in her article, 'Drug Companies and Doctors: A Story of Corruption', for the *New York Review of Books*, when she says,

> *'It is simply no longer possible to believe much of the clinical research that is published, or to rely on the judgment of trusted physicians or authoritative medical guidelines. I take no pleasure in this conclusion, which I reached slowly and reluctantly over my two decades as an editor ...'*

It's common knowledge today that the pharmaceutical industry is a multi-trillion dollar industry that wields enormous power within the world of medicine. Many cures or treatment systems which cannot be patented by the pharmaceutical giants are frequently deemed to be in opposition to their interests, and will often face a one-sided legal battle, from which, inevitably, there is only one winner.

Please do not misunderstand me – I am not saying that you should avoid traditional medicine, nor that 'alternative' remedies always work. What I am saying is that it will serve you to be circumspect about what you assume to be true, based on questionable propaganda. Certainly, no treatment should be excluded from consideration because it's not understood by, or is not palatable to, mainstream thinking.

An Holistic Approach

There is an abundance of negative research regarding practices such as yoga, meditation, Chinese medicine, homeopathy and many others. Yet, in my view, any treatment system or health-giving practice (ancient or modern) can be harmful if not practiced under guidance, and in such a way that it's personalised to an individual.

I also feel that it's a little ignorant to dismiss practices such as Chinese medicine, yoga and Ayurveda when they've been around for many thousands of years, and their efficacy, when practiced correctly, is beyond doubt. For example, the Chinese are 17 times less likely to get heart disease, and five times less likely to get breast cancer than Americans (www.doctorshealthpress.com/landingpages/chgs29).

Holistic, *natural* healing systems which have grown out of ancient wisdom have a huge amount to offer in terms of prevention of stress, chronic health problems and disease, since their remit is to heal the individual on all levels. For example, the approach of the 'Simonton Method' in the cure of cancer is to embrace a patient's beliefs, attitudes and lifestyle choices, as well as their spiritual and psychological perspectives, since these have been proven to dramatically affect the course of a disease.

The internet is awash with information about natural remedies and cures, such as turmeric, garlic, marijuana extract and many more. Indeed, Rosie Walford's article on 'bio prospecting' demonstrates the importance of ancient, tribal wisdom:

> *'"Primitive" medicinal systems hold secrets to new and effective cures. Drug companies are most interested to discover which plants indigenous medicine men are using, having realized that following a shaman increases the screening hit rate by a staggering 60 per cent.'*[12]

Wayne Dyer, Chris Wark and Francisco all embraced an holistic approach to healing which recognized the layers of their being. Most of all, they realized that they needed to take charge of their own health and healing, not only so that they could be responsible for the decisions which they took, but also in the realization of their significant role in the healing process.

Integrative Medicine

Integrative medicine is the combination of complementary and alternative medicine (CAM), and modern, western medicine. Just as the human being is comprised of many bodies or layers, so too health, healing and wellbeing are comprised of many bodies of knowledge.

Integrative medicine, or integrative healthcare, has been popularized by, among others, Deepak Chopra, Prince Charles and Dr Andrew Weil. High-profile individuals such as these believe that patients should at least supplement their western medicine with alternative therapies, and in some cases, opt solely for a personalized program focusing on nutrition, herbal remedies, meditation and other 'alternative' strategies.

Imagine the incredible possibilities of the co-operation between all the brilliant minds, bodies of knowledge and systems within the entire field of healthcare, medicine and holistic wellbeing:

Western (allopathic) doctors with their skills in examination and diagnosis, and holistic doctors and complementary therapists with their perspective of seeing the 'whole' of the picture, and having a concern for prevention above all else. This way, the whole human being is being considered – from superficial symptoms through to essential, root causes. What if there was a simple policy of advocating 'whatever works', as determined by a new system of objective testing:

**The propagation of treatments and practices that are proven
to work, regardless of the reasons why, and in spite of the
positive or negative commercial implications**

I was particularly influenced in this section of the book by my good friends Dr Shikha and her partner Matthias. Several years ago, I was advised to go and see Dr Shikha about a persistent, non-acute issue that had troubled me for many years (which I just referred to in the 'Self-healing' section). On entering the Healthy Healing Clinic in Goa, I had a minor epiphany, since I realized that I was looking at the future of clinical medicine.

Dr Shikha was trained in western medicine, but after growing frustrated with its lack of results in treating chronic illness, she set about re-training herself as an holistic, or integrative, doctor. Her old clinic (recently relocated nearby) where I saw her was small and humble, but she was inspiring and very much alive.

What I experienced under her care was an altogether different approach to chronic sickness, prevention and healing. In short, I felt totally 'heard', on all levels of my being. My issue has dropped away, and quite apart from the incredible healing systems that she uses (such as ozone therapy, chelation, colon hydrotherapy and platelet-rich plasma) I have learnt a huge amount about the doctor–patient relationship, as well as my role in the healing process.

Health and healing are a deeply personal matter, unique to each one of us. What we require to prevent ill-health or to heal ourselves once it befalls us, and how this is influenced by our quality of mind, means that generalizing the diagnostic and treatment processes is inefficient at best.

A clear picture of health and healing has to reach far deeper than the western clinical model normally allows for, or its prescriptions will frequently only be treating the superficial symptoms. As Hippocrates said:

'It's more important to know what sort of person has a disease, than to know what sort of disease a person has.'

As well as considering the patient as a unique individual, integrative medicine recognizes that whilst the skill and empathy of the practitioner, as well as the efficacy of their system, are extremely valuable in the healing process, the role of the patient must also be encouraged and supported. Good health and healthy healing require that we as individuals are empowered to be responsible for ourselves.

This means being given sufficient information regarding any disease or treatment, and also being encouraged to research and 'get involved'. To this end, when we do consult doctors and therapists, a 'lifestyle program' to take home and integrate into our daily lives would seem to me to be key to the efficacy and integrity of any treatment or practice. The rational for any such program might be:

How do we encourage the patient/client to relax, and empower them to become involved in their own healing process, so that their natural healing capacity is catalyzed?

Traditional, western medicine encourages a culture of 'listening exclusively to the expert'. This often involves popping pills or taking medicine in the quantity, and at the times, that we are told to. If this is the full extent of the treatment process, then it's incredibly disempowering. If we're encouraged to delegate our responsibility in this way, we numb our body-mind, and therefore stop trusting ourselves to know what is best. By this, I don't mean to suggest that we know better than the expert, but rather that we have the innate ability to realize what resonates with us as to the right course of action for our healing.

The benefits of integrating conventional medicine and alternative healthcare based on ancient and modern holistic wisdom are beyond doubt. Herein there's the possibility for what I spoke of a moment ago in 'Miracle Cures', which is that of combining a positive quality of mind with an assortment of carefully chosen healing modalities. In many cases, this has proven to be the best way to optimize the healing process, and fortunately we can see an increasing number of examples of integrative medical care across the globe today.

I recently came across a great example of integrative medicine in the form of a video called 'Back In the Ring' (http://backinthering.com). This initiative started in Norway as an experimental program to prove that yoga can help people with heroin addiction 'get their lives back', and be reintegrated into society. Their 'treatment' included a period of time in an intensive yoga environment in India, with physical, emotional and mental healing aspects to it, whilst still taking their medication.

Whatever the future might hold, it seems clear that modern, western medicine, though vital, will play a lesser role for those of us who become responsible for our own wellbeing. In so doing, we firmly embrace the possibility for prevention and healing, through committing to being in our *natural* state as often as we can, and therefore adopting healthy beliefs and lifestyle choices.

Quite apart from the personal benefits to ourselves, and the positive impact that we will be having on others, this will also increasingly lighten the load on traditional healthcare services.

If you have a story about integrative medical care, or anything else relating to this section of the book, then I would love to hear from you. Please use the details at the end of the book to contact me.

Validation of the Complementary Realm

Although certain holistic practices have been embraced by mainstream medicine, there is a lack of clear, validated research material supporting the field of CAM, which makes it very easy for cynics to be dismissive.

Before modern, western medicine willingly opens its arms to embrace the possibility of integrative medicine, there will need to be a huge, concerted effort involving many practitioners, clinics, centers and certifying bodies, in order to bring some unity to this highly fragmented realm. Whilst this sprawling field of wisdom has individual, representative bodies, it is largely unregulated. Although I have occasionally referred to it as CAM, many of these healing systems have been around for thousands of years – it's therefore rather disparaging to refer to them merely as 'complementary' and 'alternative'.

Perhaps there should be a new name for this vast realm of practices and systems. What about Holistic and Natural Heathcare – HNH?

There are literally hundreds of HNH sites out there on the WWW, and thousands more blogs, forums, and associated magazines and portals of valuable information. Yet it's immensely difficult to find cohesion of viewpoint, and to know what to trust. Because of this, when we fall sick, and are seeking an alternative to mainstream medicine, the most common step that we take is to Google our 'issue'. This is largely hit-and-miss, and is an altogether unsatisfactory solution.

Where are the respected industry bodies which can provide solid, scientific validation?

In fairness, the sheer size of this body of wisdom is daunting. Yet, perhaps the co-creation of an authoritative platform across the full spectrum of HNH would be a great vision for us to realize. A platform which offers a breadth of information and guidance, and, through members' interaction, produces a consensus about what works. I shall say more about this in the final section of the book. Again, I would love to hear from you in regards to this matter.

Practical Exercise

Please answer the following questions. Before you begin, first SOAR.

- How do I feel about traditional, western clinical medicine (primary healthcare)?
- What does 'holistic approach' mean to me?
- Do I sense that ancient wisdom and a more holistic approach are gaining credence today?
- Do I feel that this is a good thing, and if so, why?
- Have I experienced integrative medicine or HNH?
- If so, was my experience positive?
- Do I think it's important to raise awareness for HNH practices?
- Would I value an initiative which made it easier for me to access HNH practices?
- Would I like to know more about individual HNH practices?

Notes

1. 'These Four Beliefs Defy Modern Science...', Mercola.com, http://articles.mercola.com/sites/articles/archive/2009/09/15/these-four-beliefs-defy-modern-science.aspx.
2. Johann Hari, 'The Likely Cause of Addiction Has Been Discovered, and it is Not What You Think', Huffington Post, www.huffingtonpost.com/johann-hari/the-real-cause-of-addicti_b_6506936.html.
3. Dr Frank Lipman, '2 Questions to Ask That Are More Important Than a Diagnosis' Huffington Post, www.huffingtonpost.com/dr-frank-lipman/2-questions-to-ask-that-a_b_220293.html.
4. Chris Bell, *The Telegraph*, 16 October 2013.
5. Dr Rupert Sheldrake, quoted in 'Integrative Medicine and Medical Qigong Therapy', www.qigonginstitute.org/html/advertising/qigong_therapyaviva.php.
6. David Hamilton, 'The Amazing Power of the Placebo', David R Hamilton PhD website, http://drdavidhamilton.com/the-amazing-power-of-the-placebo.
7. David Hamilton, 'The Amazing Power of the Placebo', David R Hamilton PhD website, http://drdavidhamilton.com/the-amazing-power-of-the-placebo-2.
8. Including your choice of healer/practitioner/doctor, and the treatment process.
9. 'Chris Beat Cancer', blog, www.chrisbeatcancer.com.
10. Ben Goldacre, 'What Doctors Don't Know About the Drugs They Prescribe', TED, www.ted.com/talks ben_goldacre_what_doctors_don_t_know_about_the_drugs_they_prescribe?language=en.
11. Dr Marcia Agnell is also the author of *The Truth About the Drug Companies: How They Deceive Us and What to Do About It*.
12. Rosie Walford Telegraph Magazine, www.e-o-n.org/rosiewalford/bioprospect_teleg.htm.

Summary Chapter 6

Taking Responsibility For Your Sickness And Healing

This chapter explored the role that you play in your own healing, according to your quality of mind and therefore also your lifestyle choices. As Dr Mercola said:

'If your thoughts and emotions play such a significant role in modifying your biology and your health (and I believe they do), then treating your emotions becomes an essential part of optimal health.'

1. What is Chronic Disease?

Chronic disease includes stress and all other diseases which persist for a prolonged period of time. Ancient sages realized that our body-mind operates in much the same way as a river – when it's not polluted, it can effectively deal with most unwanted intruders by virtue of our immune system:

It is the health of your inner environment (the field) which determines the effect that outside factors such as germs and your surroundings will have on your physical being

- *Symptoms are the language of the body* – These visible 'hot spots' are not a problem, but a warning of an underlying issue. Stress and disease can be seen as an invitation for heightened awareness, and symptoms may be embraced with gratitude rather than fear.

- *The roots of stress and chronic disease* – Ancient tribal medicine men and women realized the connection between emotions, state of mind, and the way in which villagers became sick. They viewed unhappiness and sickness as an undernourishment of the human spirit, or a lack of joy and inner peace.

- *Total load* – This refers to the sum total of all those factors which might impair your wellbeing.

2. *Embracing Your Role in Your Own Healing*

Your mental and emotional states are key to your healing because of the way in which they impact upon your subconscious mind and the systems of your body.

- *The Placebo Effect (Your Doctor Within)* – At least one-third of all healing, including drugs, surgery and other allopathic interventions, has nothing to do with the process, but has to do with the body's self-healing capacity.

- *Self-healing* – The mind is not separate from the body – hence why I refer to them as body-mind. Your role in your own healing is two-fold:

  - *Natural* Quality of Mind – Wake Up and SOAR and the 10 Mantras
  - Supportive Lifestyle Choices – Your Personal Support System

- *Miracle Cures* – When a person actively engages in their own healing process, they invite life to support them in every way possible. There are never any guarantees, since life is a mystery, but when a range of carefully considered elements are combined – positive quality of mind, loving surroundings and the right mix of healing processes – then magic is possible.

3. A More Integrated Approach to Medicine

- *The Dawn of a New Approach to Healing and Medicine* – The complementary and alternative medical (CAM) industry is burgeoning, and there's a growing awareness that prevention is better than cure. We're beginning to see practices such as yoga therapy, acupuncture, herbal medicine, myriad forms of massage and so on entering mainstream medicine. Healing is beginning to be understood as a return to optimal wellbeing on all levels, rather than curing apparent problems.

- *Modern Western Medicine* – There have been miraculous advances, particularly in the area of 'acute medicine', but the unwillingness to embrace an holistic approach means that it's often ineffective in dealing with stress and chronic disease, and healing the totality of the problem.

- *An Holistic Approach* – Holistic, *natural* healing systems which have grown out of ancient wisdom have a huge amount to offer in terms of prevention of stress, chronic health problems and disease. These systems recognize that our beliefs, attitudes, lifestyle choices, and spiritual and psychological perspectives can dramatically affect our health, the course of our disease and our overall wellbeing.

- *Integrative Medicine* – This is the combination of complementary and alternative medicine (CAM), and modern, western medicine. As well as considering the patient as a unique individual, integrative medicine recognizes that the role of the patient must be encouraged and supported, and that there may well be the need for a multi-faceted healing process.

- *Validation of the Complementary Realm* – There is a lack of clear, validated research material supporting the field of CAM. Imagine the co-creation of an authoritative platform with a breadth of information, guidance and consensus about what works. Perhaps we could call this vast realm Holistic and Natural Healthcare (HNH)

Part 3

The Third Key

Pursue Your Dreams

'Fly'

Part 1 provides a tool – Wake Up and SOAR – for addressing the essential problem that we all face as human beings – the *normal* state of mind. This tool allows you to relax and return to your *natural* state at will. I have also suggested the 10 Mantras as additional mini-meditations, which help you to embrace acceptance – the essence of SOAR and inviting your *natural* quality of mind.

Part 2 shows you that you are attracting your life towards you, and you must therefore take responsibility for your own wellbeing and nurture yourself. When you know how to calm your mind, and you use your Personal Support System, you can optimize your own wellbeing, and support your own healing.

Part 3 is about realizing that once you know how to calm your mind, and you have a supportive lifestyle, you have a stable base with which to pursue your dreams and fly. When you calmly pursue your heartfelt desires, you unleash your creative fire and come alive. This both feeds you, and also allows you to impact positively upon others. This is precisely how you play your role in the bigger picture of life, and is what I call the Law Of Magic – the Third Tool. There are two components to this tool –

- Pursuing your heartfelt desires feeds you

- Your coming alive serves others

'DREAMS OF FLYING'

The images within my dream are always more or less the same. I am walking along the pavement, often close to my childhood home in Wimbledon, when I will spontaneously 'lift off' into the air. I soar above the people walking on the pavement, and effortlessly fly around, and between, buildings and trees. I always have the feeling of deep relaxation and incredible freedom. I am unlimited, and full of loving gratitude for this.

Sometimes my trips are quite short and close to the ground, and at other times I fly great distances. When I first started to have these dreams, I was surprised each time I took off and realized that I could fly. After some years, though, I grew accustomed to my extraordinary talent; nonetheless, the sensation was just as euphoric and beautiful.

These dreams have been extremely powerful for me. The imagery of flying is particularly potent, since it alludes to a 'super-power' which enables me to take off and SOAR beyond normal earthly limitations. What is key to the experience, I feel, is that it is utterly effortless. In fact I feel like I'm doing what I'm most naturally designed to do.

Even though the dreams are experienced whilst asleep, I have begun to be able to observe my dream as it is going on, and subtly direct it. Instead of allowing myself to fall into 'wanting to impress people' with my feats of flying I choose to remain calm and to spread my positive vibration. What I've learnt is that

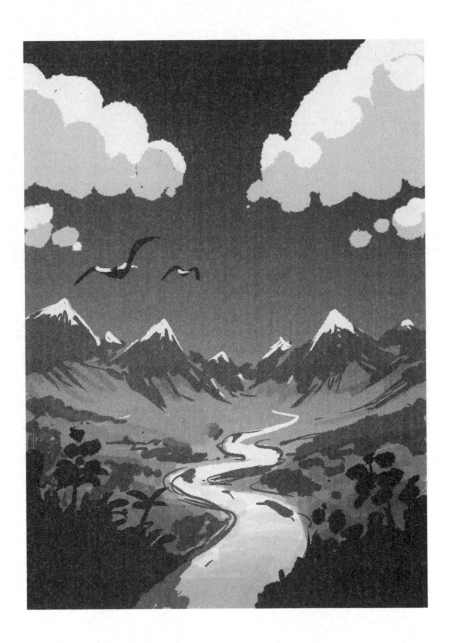

even when I'm riding the waves of my natural frame of mind – SOARing – if I don't remain vigilant, I can easily slide back towards my normal, egocentric frame of mind.

I've come to realize that my ability to 'take off and fly' allows me to impact positively upon others. It's as if their inner, creative fire is enlivened by my aliveness, and they experience their own sense of 'flying'. Of course I've also recognized that what I've experienced within the dream is a wonderful metaphor for how I can live my daily life.

There is nothing more incredible than sensing just how much life wants you to flourish. I have always been full of dreams, and fairly confident about pursuing them. But like everyone else, I've had my fair share of failures. Those life situations which knock you flat, and for a period of time make you wonder if you will ever recover. So when I see that life is clearly telling me that I am capable of so much more than just 'normal', this is deeply empowering.

My dreams of taking off and flying are life talking to me, gently urging me to realize that I can fly – and that this is absolutely natural. I have had dreams of flying since I was a kid. However, there was a period in my early thirties, around the time that I had the inner voice saying 'slow down', that these dreams became more regular and deeply impacting.

These dreams have also woven themselves into the fabric of this book, without me having realized it. It's only on reflection that I see this. Life is a magical mystery tour, an opportunity to 'take off and fly'. But we can only know this when we drop the idea that we can control life. This is the dichotomy of life. On the one hand, I am a sentient human being making choices; but at a far deeper level, I am a vessel through which life's energy courses. The more that my heart and mind are open, the more effortless and beautiful the journey.

A short time ago, after one such dream, I wrote the following:

THE MAGIC CARPET RIDE

Life force
life's vital energy
courses through each of us
inviting us on her magic carpet ride
providing us with precisely what we require
in the perfect measure, embracing us all, and urging us
to pursue our heartfelt desires so that we might love ourselves
and all that surrounds us, and experience the simple joy of being alive.
Life empowers us all with the freedom to feel fully alive, happy and healthy
inspired by our purpose and dreams, and passionately pursuing
those dreams with reckless abandon and limitless creativity
living with wonder and innocence and learning how to
plunge ever deeper into loving and being loved
and then sharing this joy and wellbeing
with all of our brothers and sisters
knowing that at depth
we are all one –
we are life
itself

Chapter 7

The Law of Magic (Part 1)
Pursuing Your Heartfelt Desires Feeds You

The Law of Magic (Part 1)

So there it is, my recurring dreams of flying are about SOARing.

'Take off and fly' is a precise reflection of Wake Up and SOAR; the associated feelings of effortlessness, deep relaxation and freedom are a message that I am unlimited, so long as I am flying – in my *natural* quality of mind.

Part of the purpose of this book is to encourage you to see that you and I are, at source, the same. We have the same capacity to tame our lake monster and therefore create compelling lives. We are all capable of climbing aboard our own private magic carpet and SOARing. This is our birthright. How effectively we do this is dependent upon the extent to which we invite, and surf, our *natural* quality of mind.

So now it's time to learn to fly. Or, better said, it's now time to remember that you already know how to fly. By 'fly', I mean sensing your deepest dreams, 'and passionately pursuing those dreams with reckless abandon and limitless creativity'.

In my experience, if you don't honor what is there in your heart and mind, and it's something that you truly want, then you are doing yourself and those around you a great disservice. Your greatest gift to yourself, and to those around you whom you love, is to be happy and well.

In Chapter 4, 'The Law of Karma: You Attract Your Life Towards You', we saw that you're attracting your life according to your thought vibrations. But does this mean that you can attract into your life anything that you want?

There are books and self-help programs which state categorically that 'You can have, be and do anything that you want.' In fact there has been something of an epidemic of this idea sweeping the world over the last few years. Whilst in theory this may seem true, it is overly simplistic, since it doesn't take account of the indescribable complexity of life.

It obviously isn't true to say that you are so much in control of life that you can ask anything of her, and then expect her to produce this for you, let alone claim to have any idea about when this will come to pass. This belief, or hope, arises from a *normal* state of mind. Dilip had expectations of life which were simply unrealistic –

The Law of Magic (Part 1)

'Dilip was less surrendered to the majesty of Mother Nature, believing that life was cheating him of what he really deserved – an easy life, with lots of money ...'

Life is a mystery. You can't say a few affirmations, and simply expect that you will be adorned with riches, it doesn't work that way. I would therefore prefer to say that when you are calm (*natural* quality of mind), you are able to intuit and feel what you truly desire – what makes your heart sing. You can then gently ask life to support you in manifesting what it is that you truly, deeply desire.

Sometimes, all that you can do is to stay open for the possibility of your deepest desire to become reality. For example, if you wish to attract a soul-mate into your life. At other times, you might need to embark upon a creative project, where you take consistent, focused action in order to pursue your heartfelt goal. Whichever the case, it is your awareness of what it is that you truly desire, and your clarity of intention, which cause you to unleash your creative fire and invite the Law of Magic.

If you sense what you truly desire, and you calmly set your intention upon this, then you unleash your creative fire and you invite[1] what you truly desire into reality. This feeds you deeply.

This is Part 1 of the Law of Magic.

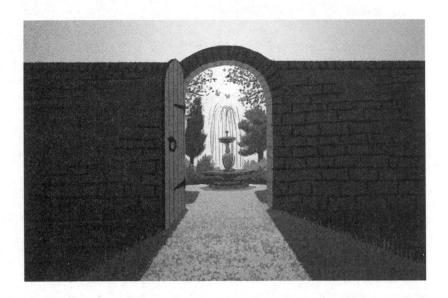

Unleashing Your Creative Fire

When you calmly pursue your heartfelt desires, you unleash your creative fire, which means that you come alive. If your heartfelt desire requires some form of creative expression, then, more than likely, unleashing your creative fire will encompass knowing what your unique talents are, and embracing what you most love to do. This yields an endless reserve of creativity and passion, and you have the magical ingredients for loving your life.

It all begins with knowing how to tame your lake monster, and therefore having a calm mind. When your mind is still, and the lake monster is quiet, what lies at depth is revealed – 'a kaleidoscope of color with a myriad of indescribably beautiful reflections'. In other words, when your mind is calm, you sense what it is that you truly desire, and you are able to use the law of attraction in the most magical way – a powerful, karmic chain of events is set into motion.

Because you are calm, you become clear about what you truly want – your heartfelt desire, which you can therefore develop into a clear purpose ...

With clarity of purpose, you are inspired to create a plan to realize your dream, which you can then act upon with a laser-like focus ...

So long as you remain focused without becoming obsessed (stressed), you are constantly inviting life's support, and you access all the wisdom, love, creative energy and playfulness that you require to pursue your dream.

So there are three parts to the Law of Magic (Part 1). The first involves developing a clear vision of what it is that you wish to make happen; the second involves the plan, and taking action upon that plan; and the third requires that you stay relaxed and grounded, so that you're inviting life's support and you are therefore enjoying the journey:

1   Envisioning
•   Heartfelt Desire – the Why
•   Clarity of Purpose – the What

2   Taking Action
•   The Plan – the How
•   Focused Action – the Action

3   Inviting Life's Support

This section of the book will be that much more productive if you have some particular dream, project or goal in mind. So please take a moment to consider this, and use your journal to makes notes as you read through this section. It's so often the case that in stepping out from your 'comfort zone', the ideas and clarity will begin to flow. Life is always walking towards you, but she needs you to meet her halfway.

1. Envisioning

Heartfelt Desire – the Why

Your heartfelt desire is the essence of your dream or goal. This is the most magical ingredient which you bring to the table, because all else springs forth from this. If you don't have the desire to dream, and to imagine beautiful possibilities for yourself, then what can you hope to achieve? Equally, if you are forever vacillating in your wants and desires, what can life do?

But if you connect with your heartfelt desires and stay focused, then magic is possible, and life becomes the creative endeavor that it is meant to be. This is using the law of attraction in its most beautiful and potent form.

What would life be without heartfelt dreams? What caused us to jump out of bed when we were young, innocent children? And why shouldn't we remain innocent, and passionate about our dreams and deepest desires?

Please take a moment to SOAR. How does it make you feel?

When you SOAR, this means to a limitless depth. And by depth, I don't mean within your body — which is, of course, limited. I mean up and outwards, to the furthest reaches of the known Universe.

This is why the expression 'falling in love', is such a poor reflection of something so indescribably wonderful. No wonder it is a misunderstood phenomenon. When you are discovering your depth of love for another person, a project or whatever it might be, you are anything but 'falling'. You are very definitely rising, or SOARing in love. As I said in the 10 Mantras:

'Love is life's omnipotent force causing your being to expand upwards and outwards, so that you merge with life itself.'

Isn't this true? When you are experiencing those incomparable feelings of being in love, aren't you surfing on a magic carpet above and beyond worldly troubles?

When you are in touch with your heartfelt desires, regarding a goal or project, it's similar to being in love. I become in love with most of my projects. If I don't feel the love flowing through me, then I don't bother to begin, or continue. Yes, for sure, there are difficult moments, just as with friendships and love relationships, but if the love is not able to flow, then the Why is not strong enough. I pursue what I love. Anything less would be like hard work.

I fully acknowledge that the mundane practicalities of life will often seem to limit our ability to pursue our dreams.

But is this really true, or is it a cop-out?

I believe that whatever it is that you truly want is there in your field of possibility. It's what you're meant to pursue. If you change your mind, and go off the idea, then that's something else. Perhaps it wasn't truly heartfelt after all, or life's mysterious ways sent you a curve ball. But please don't make excuses about dreams that were unobtainable. If you truly want it, from the depth of your being, then go for it!

Whatever it is that you truly want is what causes you to feel fully alive and be in the flow of life. This means that because of the passion and clarity with which you act, even when you face challenges, they are surmounted as if you're supported by outside forces (which is precisely so).

I like to ask people about their dreams, and how they would like to be living their lives. I am frequently surprised to hear people say, 'I haven't really given that much thought.' Or they mention something that they love to do, and after their eyes have temporarily lit up, they quickly add, 'But I can't make a living from that because ...'

It is my observation that many people believe in some way that they are not worthy of their dreams. They believe that a deeply fulfilling life, manifesting one's dreams, is for others. When you live with such resignation, you ask life to support you in your belief that you are not worthy of doing what you love.

Bronnie Ware, the palliative nurse that I spoke of before, said this on the subject of 'the most common regret' of the dying:

'Most people had not honored even a half of their dreams and had to die knowing that it was due to choices they had made, or not made. Health brings a freedom very few realize, until they no longer have it.'²

What Makes Your Heart Sing?

This is a question that I frequently ask people when we're discussing dreams and goals. I also ask this of people when they are applying for a job at Ashiyana, but I might rephrase it as 'What do you love to do?'

It's an important question, because when most people compare their answer with what they spend the majority of their time doing, there is normally a poor correlation.

So please consider this question for a moment, and then write down your thoughts in your journal:

'What makes your heart sing?'

Ok, now let's take a good look at your life and see just how much time and energy you give to what it is that you most love to do. Give it a percentage – this per cent of my waking day I spend doing what I most love to do.

There's no wrong or right here. It's for you to assess how you feel about this percentage. So take a moment, and SOAR.

Now, with a calm mind, how do you feel about the time and energy that you give to what you most love to do?

It can be helpful to remember that your body-mind 'vehicle' has an expiry date, as this focuses your mind on the need to live your dreams before it's too late. In the Buddhist tradition of Bhutan, the Bhutanese people practice 'awareness of death', five times a day. They believe that regularly contemplating their mortality causes them to appreciate life whilst they are still alive. It's worth remembering that this is the country whose leader created the concept of 'gross national happiness'. Whatever it is that makes your heart sing is precisely what will enable you to unleash your creative fire. This is your most potent Why. So take the time to consider carefully what you truly desire.

Once again, let me state clearly that what I am referring to has nothing to do with the idea: 'You can have, be and do anything that you want'! By now I am pretty sure that you can sense how this way of thinking emanates from a programed, *normal* state of mind. It's simply not true. Not because life limits you in what you can achieve. It's much more basic than that. It's not true, because it's not what you truly want!

When you have a heartfelt desire for something, it's because it's already within your field of possibility – a reality in its unmanifest form (invisible field of life), waiting to be brought into 'manifest' reality (physical form).

The Law of Magic, therefore, is not about you embarking upon an egoistic mission to 'have, be and do' whatever you might randomly desire. This Law requires only that you slow down, and sense deeply what wants to happen. This means an awareness of your inner realm of stillness, which necessitates a commitment to Wake Up and SOAR.

The Law Of Magic has no time for superficial whims. Wanting to get rich, or develop a 'beach-fit body' are likely to be unfulfilling endeavors for most of us. Not because we can't achieve them, but because they arise from a *normal* quality of mind, and yield the 'superficial blip of calm and happiness'.

If you want to love your life, and be close friends with the Law of Magic, then stay focused on 'What makes my heart sing?'

The Power of Intention

Be honest with yourself about what you truly love to do, and don't procrastinate in your pursuit of your dreams. The Law of Magic begins with dreaming. What you're dreaming about is unimportant to life: she pays close attention to the vibration of your intention – your willingness to pursue your heartfelt desire.

It's not important how big or small your vision, what matters is your intention to take full responsibility for your part in the realization of it

Be sure that you are not somehow limiting yourself, through fear of failure, or apathy, or other *normal* qualities of mind. It's a sad but utterly accurate observation that if you don't change your direction, you will end up precisely where you're heading; and that may not be very satisfying.

If you are not overflowing with passion about some great purpose, then please don't worry.

Always remember that life is a mystery – there are no 'should's' and 'shouldn't's' within a *natural* quality of mind. If you are easily able to connect with your passion then that's great. If not that's also fine, just remember the eighth of the 10 Mantras – be patient. When the moment is right for you to realize a wonderful objective and pursue your heartfelt desires, you will be the first to know.

So be patient until you discover what stirs your soul, and then let your imagination run wild, exploring all those dreams which you might previously have dismissed as unattainable. Life is sitting in readiness for you to declare what it is you feel most passionately about. Once you've declared this inwardly, with a clear, calm voice, life commands her tribe of aids to assist you in your pursuit of your dreams. She makes no promises about the outcome, but she lovingly embraces your intention.

Passing dreams are not enough – they are like impotent whims. When your desires are superficial, you are either unlikely to achieve them, or they will yield no real fulfillment. So you must have the intention to sense what you deeply desire, and then have the courage to take action. There are no prizes for having great ideas, nor for imagining great undertakings. Life rewards the brave!

Please remember – you are the master of your life experience – so if you are not choosing your pathway through envisioning the life that you truly want to be living, then your unconscious thoughts (*normal* state) will be creating a trajectory regardless.

Clarity of Purpose – the What

Clarity of purpose is your heartfelt desire expressed as a clear objective, this makes it more compelling and easier to envision.

When you know Why you are doing something, and What that is going to look like, you have an abundance of inspiration and energy with which to act. This kind of 'engagement' with what you are doing invites your *natural* quality of mind, and you are far more likely to realize your vision.

Humans flourish when they have purpose, and they tend to suffer when they are idle or directionless. If you imagine yourself on a deserted island, you might easily visualize the need for a purpose of some sort or another to stave off boredom and give some meaning to your life.

It may be that you imagine foraging for food and collecting rainwater, or perhaps maintaining your grass-roofed, bamboo dwelling. Whatever it is, whether essential and practical, or more for pleasure, there will be the desire for a daily purpose.

At a basic level, you are designed to survive, procreate, love, pursue pleasure and avoid pain – these are your base instincts. Given your sophisticated human mind, though, you can evolve from this primal state into living your life with a far deeper purpose.

For many people in today's world, notions of purpose will tend to revolve strongly around work and traditional ideas about success. Work is the principle role that brings income, and it occupies much of your time during the week. It's also one of the most obvious measures of how you are performing in life, as perceived by your peers, friends and family.

Because of this, 'success' at work may easily become the principle determinant of your sense of fulfillment. Accordingly, ambition, recognition, promotion and financial success are highly prized.

But purpose is not a tool for driving yourself forward in order to have and consume more. Rather it is a beautiful inner guidance system that allows you to stay focused on what is really important for you in your life.

Clarity of purpose, therefore, means having a clear picture of what you want to achieve. A clear What, backed by a compelling Why, means that your focus will be strong, you will be guided by universal wisdom, and you will have an abundance of energy and resolve you can draw upon.

'When you are inspired by some great purpose, some extraordinary project, all your thoughts break their bonds: Your mind transcends limitations, your consciousness expands in every direction, and you find yourself in a new, great and wonderful world. Dormant forces, faculties and talents become alive, and you discover yourself to be a greater person by far than you ever dreamed yourself to be.' Patanjali

Whatever it is you chose as your dream, goal or project at the beginning of this section, how clear are you about what you want? Can you easily define it? What is your 'elevator pitch' – if you met someone in a lift/elevator, and had to explain your dream, goal or project to them, what would you say in a few words?

It may be that you have a particular project in mind, or perhaps a more abstract purpose. You might be temporarily doing something that you are not so keen on, in the knowledge that it serves a longer-term purpose of saving money to travel or start your own business. You may be able to clearly define what your overriding life mission is, or maybe you are motivated by day-to-day objectives. Perhaps you have the intention of growing and maturing as a person.

No one person's purpose is more valid than another's, since we are each here to fulfill our own unique life purpose. Whatever it is that creates a strong engagement with what you are doing invites your *natural* quality of mind, and this is the key to maintaining focus.

When you have clarity of purpose, and you consistently follow your heartfelt desires and dreams, you are able to re-write the 'hard-wired' programing accumulated over a lifetime. Even the particular circumstances – the synchronicity – that might prevail for a specific instance of success are inherent within anything that is driven by heartfelt desire and clarity of purpose.

Heartfelt implies that you are sensing what life is calling for you to do, and in situations such as these life provides you with whatever exceptional circumstances are required for you to succeed. 'Luck' is not a random phenomenon. It has been attracted by everything that you have ever thought, said and done during this lifetime, and perhaps past lifetimes also. The Law of Karma is always operating.

So, clarity of purpose means clarifying your Why, so that it becomes a clear purpose. For example, if your Why is that you are passionate about singing, you may also want to make some money from this. Perhaps you have a vision of doing gigs in your local area:

- Heartfelt Desire – the Why: to sing
- Clarity of Purpose – the What: to gig in your local area

So what you're now able to envision is – 'I want to get gigs in my local area, because I love to sing.'

What you're envisioning then, your Why and your What, needs to be a compelling purpose, and this encompasses two elements – heartfelt desire and clarity of purpose. Clarity of purpose gives you direction, and heartfelt desire provides your fuel.

I strongly recommend that you begin to write down the thoughts of what you are envisioning, in the way that I have done above. Even create a 'mood board'³ if you like, with visuals that inspire you towards achieving your goal. This can be developed as you embellish it with a more detailed plan, which we are going to look at next.

2. Taking Action

The Plan – the How

Whether you are setting up a new business, looking for a new job, getting married, or simply going to the shops, it is important to have a plan of action. This plan will have a few elements to it, and the more evolved and complex the plan, the more the elements.

For example, using the previous example again – if you have a genuine passion for singing, and you would love to start off by doing gigs in your area, what is your plan to achieve this?

The following list will suffice for this example, and probably for most other endeavors. This plan is not set in stone, it will evolve, as you meet obstacles and recognize the need to adapt and adjust your thinking. It will also need to be fleshed out, and perhaps turned into a well-laid-out presentation, especially if you need to attract key team members, or investors:

1   The vision/concept (the Why and the What)

2   Your strengths/skills/loves

3   The team (if required) to complement your skills and achieve this vision

4   Research regarding demand/timing, venues, office space, job market, etc.

5   Marketing/promotion for what you will do to to promote your vision

6   Time considerations

7   Financial considerations

It's important that every time you think about your dream or project, you are excited and feel a surge of energy. The visual aspect of the mood board will help with this.

Focused Action – the Action

Action

Research demonstrates that people who have a tendency to take action are more fulfilled, since they are rewarded by their progress and are therefore propelled to do more. Over-analyzing situations tends to result in a lack of decisive action.

The hardest part of taking action is usually the first step. If you can galvanize yourself into action, through taking that first step, then in my experience life places signposts along the pathway that you need to follow. Don't procrastinate, ignorantly believing that it will be easier to take the first step tomorrow.

Be bold * Be brave * SOAR

However, action is not enough. The action you take needs to be focused. Focused on what?
Focused on your compelling purpose!

Life rewards you for the action that you take; the more that your actions are in line with your heartfelt desires, the more you invite life to support you and work her magic. Somehow it just works this way – as you learn to pursue your deepest desires, life conspires to open doors for you.

Focus

When you are calm, and you have clarity of purpose, you will easily stay focused. If your Why, What and How are clear and compelling, then you will naturally develop a laser-like focus. This focus will inspire you to keep taking action.

When you have a laser-like focus, your frequency of vibration is crystal clear and you are using the law of attraction in its most potent form. This will ensure that you invite the Law of Magic to the party!

Let me exemplify this with the tool SOAR, and how it was 'born':

Over the years, I have evolved my own way of calming my mind, which has been deeply informed by my time with Satyananda.

Whilst writing this book, over a period of months, I would regularly stop what I was doing and be still for a few moments. Often, I would sit with my eyes closed, observing what was going on inside. In other words, I paid attention to what was arising within my body-mind. I ignored everything that was happening around me, and focused my attention towards the depth of my being.

In this way, I broke down the key elements of what I was naturally doing to calm my mind. It was this:

- Slowing everything down (preferably sitting down and closing my eyes)
- Observing inwardly and connecting with my breath
- Noticing what was arising without attaching to it – Accepting
- As I stayed there observing, I would grow more relaxed – Relaxing

This became:

SOAR

S – Slow down (sit down and close your eyes if possible)
O – Observe inwardly and connect with your breathing
A – Accept all that is arising without judgment or resistance
R – Relax deeply and sense your inner peace of being

So a powerful tool was born whilst I was pursuing my heartfelt desire to write this book – taking action in a highly focused way. The 10 Mantras arose in much the same way.

Wake Up and SOAR has provided me with a tool which I can apply to any life situation. Please note, the key here is applying the tool – taking action! Thinking about the tool is useless, you need to actually use it in the cut and thrust of life – when you are emotionally 'triggered'; to aid falling asleep at night; first thing in the morning – literally Wake Up and SOAR; and in any *normal* moment, when you are lost in your story.

People who love their lives and consistently feel fulfilled are not daunted by apparent failure. This requires clarity of purpose – the Why. From one perspective, my life has been an unending catalogue of mistakes and failures. What has enabled me to succeed in realizing many of my dreams, though, is my focus, which has enabled me to get back up after a fall, and keep moving forward.

True fulfillment, as opposed to a 'temporary blip of calm and happiness', is not about reaching the end of an adventure, but rather having the wisdom to know that there will be highs and lows along the way, and yet remaining steadfast in your pursuit of what you truly desire.

Vigilance

I would like to highlight something that I said in the 'Dreams of Flying' story:

> *'What I've learnt is that even when I'm riding the waves*
> *of my natural frame of mind – SOARing – if I don't*
> *remain vigilant, I can easily slide back towards my*
> *normal, egocentric frame of mind.'*

This is an important realization. When you are in your *natural* state of mind (as I am, predominantly, in my dreams), you can easily fall back into a *normal* state of mind. This is fine and human. You don't need to change.

But, and it's a very big BUT – you do need to remain vigilant.

Vigilance is akin to focus, though it specifically refers to watching out for potential difficulties. SOARing, and living from your *natural*, awakened quality of mind requires that you are attentive to your lake monster. It wasn't as simple as Arun just being lucky with his genes; and the lake didn't just happen to awaken and then tell the monster just one time to be quiet. In both instances, there was a 'powerful call of Life' – and this was responded to, vigilantly:

Arun, and the Lake, had to remain vigilant as they tamed their lake monster.

3. Inviting Life's Support

My experience is that when I am riding the waves of my heartfelt desires, I am endlessly guided and supported. This support and guidance allows me to enjoy my magic carpet ride, since it keeps inviting me towards surrendered acceptance.

In other words, when you are pursuing your heartfelt desires, so long as you don't become obsessive and therefore stressed, you are inviting your *natural* quality of mind, and the 10 Mantras are never far away.

For sure you won't be permanently experiencing your *natural* quality of mind, but when you are passionate about what you're doing, and important decisions need to made, you intuitively know what is best. And, because you trust that you will be guided, and are deeply grateful for this, you invite wise guidance into reality.

For example, in writing this book, there were endless moments of not knowing how to explain something clearly, or how to structure a chapter. But I trusted that I would work this out, and I was grateful to life when the clarity came to me. Occasionally, there were moments of frustration, but they dropped away quickly because I knew that I would be guided. Not surprisingly, the clarity would generally arise when I was deeply relaxed, such as when lying in the bath, or lying in bed after waking up.

Of course, there are going to be endless situations where guidance comes from outside of you. Perhaps you ask someone for guidance, or you read something in a book. Maybe you see something whilst walking in nature, or hear something that somebody says, and the 'penny drops'. But, if you look closely at what is actually happening here, you will see that whilst the stimuli – words, images, sounds, smells – come from outside of you, the recognition of the importance of these arises from deep within your being.

You are always being guided.
But you need to have a quiet mind to realize this.

The significance of having goals and dreams is not that you have to follow them rigidly, but that you use them as a guidance system for staying focused. In number 6 of the 10 Mantras, 'Nurture Flexibility', I said –

'You will probably have noticed that life rarely goes to plan,
hence the saying: "If you want to make the Gods laugh, tell
them your plans." If you can accept what arises, even when it's
not as you planned, or would wish it to be, then your surrender
means that you feel no tension. The ability to adapt, adjust and
accommodate for life's ways is a powerful quality.'

This is not to say that wishing to achieve your dreams is meaningless, it's more that you need to be flexible in terms of what achievement 'looks like'. Like a river, you want to reach the sea, and to do so it's wise to follow the path of least resistance, adapting and adjusting your course according to the prevailing circumstances. Pursuing your dreams this way is much easier, and a lot more fun.

For example, if I have a strong desire to build my own log cabin, then great, but precisely what it will look like, its exact dimensions, and many other details may well change. Life is about flux, impermanence, and therefore adjusting, adapting and not being rigid. Rigidity is a sure way to become stressed and disappointed.

So – envision, make appropriate plans, take the first steps, and keep taking action, always adapting and responding to the changing circumstances. The plan is there to create focus, and galvanize you into action – the exact outcome will evolve, precisely as it needs to.

When you are calm and clear about what you truly want, you are also opening your heart so that love can flow. This is an extremely important aspect of your *natural* quality of mind, because it means that you can act with patience, integrity and compassion. But as I said a moment ago, don't expect to be in a permanent state of unconditional love. Even in the case of a mother with a young baby, most of the time her love is unbounded, it springs forth naturally and in abundance ... but there will still be moments, or periods, of sadness and even depression.

So when you're riding your magic carpet, doing what you love to do, you are endlessly inviting your *natural* quality of mind, and therefore SOAR and the 10 Mantras will be close at hand.

Practical Exercise

Please answer the following questions. Before you begin, first SOAR.

- Do I believe that I have the right to pursue my heartfelt desires?
- Having read this chapter, am I becoming clearer about a dream or goal?
- If so, do I have clarity of purpose around this dream, project or goal?
- How would I describe it if asked?
- Have I started to make a plan?
- Have I already begun to take action?
- If so, am I focused in my pursuit of this plan?
- Can I feel life supporting me in my undertaking?
- Do I have trust that I will be supported?
- If I have no specific goal or dream in mind, do I feel empowered to be more productive or effective in some way in my life?
- Am I fulfilled?
- Is there perhaps something that I would love to have or do, but I doubt my worth or ability?
- If time and money were not an issue, what would I most love to be doing with my life?

Notes

1. Please note that the word invite does not mean that the outcome is guaranteed. As you will have observed, 'plans rarely go to plan'. The point is that you unleash your creative fire and come alive – this invites the magic!
2. Bronnie Ware, 'Regrets of the Dying', blog, http://bronnieware.com/regrets-of-the-dying.
3. Mood boards are used in advertising, marketing and PR as visual representations of an idea or vision. Their value lies in the fact that they are evocative. The illustrations within this book work in the same way.

Summary Chapter 7

The Law of Magic (Part 1)
Pursuing Your Heartfelt Desires Feeds You

Law of Magic (Part 1)

If you sense what you truly desire, and you calmly set your intention upon this, then you unleash your creative fire and you invite what you truly desire into reality.

Because you are calm, you become clear about what you truly want – your heartfelt desire, which you can therefore develop into a clear purpose ...

With clarity of purpose, you are inspired to create a plan to realize your dream, which you can then act upon with a laser-like focus ...

So long as you remain focused without becoming obsessed (stressed), you are constantly inviting life's support, and you access all the wisdom, love, creative energy and playfulness that you require to pursue your dream.

So there are three parts to the Law of Magic (Part 1) –

1   Envisioning

- Heartfelt Desire – the Why
- Clarity of Purpose – the What

2   Taking Action

- The Plan – the How
- Focused Action – the Action

3   Inviting Life's Support

You are always being guided.
But you need to have a quiet mind to realize this.

Chapter 8

The Law of Magic (Part 2)
Your 'Coming Alive' Serves Others

The Law of Magic (Part 1) says:

If you sense what you truly desire, and you calmly set your intention upon this, then you unleash your creative fire and you invite what you truly desire into reality. This feeds you deeply.

This then leads on to the Law of Magic (Part 2), which says:

When you unleash your creative fire through pursuing what you truly desire, you come alive, and your positive vibration touches others. Coming alive is therefore your gift to the world.

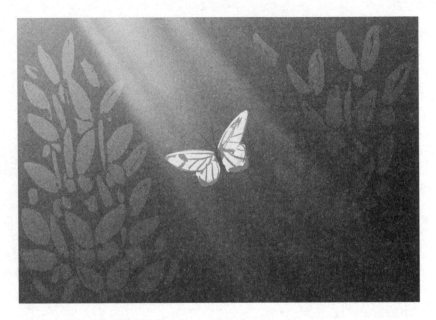

Your Vibration Matters

Have you ever considered just how much you might be benefitting others through doing what you are good at, and what you love to do?

In 'Dreams of Flying', I said:

> *'I've come to realize that my ability to 'take off and fly' is a wonderful opportunity to impact positively upon others. It's as if their inner creative fire is enlivened by my aliveness, and they experience their own sense of "flying".'*

I believe that everyone has a special talent, perhaps several if they are lucky. It really doesn't matter whether this is a talent for playing the guitar, excelling at sport, being a loving mother, listening without judgment, or having the skill and desire to be a safe bus driver.

Loving what you're doing means that you are 100 per cent alive, and you are vibrating with a positive and inspiring frequency. So doing what you love and pursuing your heartfelt desires not only feeds you, but it is also your gift to those around you.

Imagine that you're a humble bus driver, as I mentioned above, perhaps in a rural area of southern France, or Spain. If you have a passion for driving your bus, you will do so with great care for your passengers, and also for the wild animals which might run across the road in front of your bus. Your focused attention and care for what you are doing keeps others safe and affords them a pleasurable journey. Whenever you pursue what you love to do, and 'come alive', you impact positively on those around you. As I said in 'Taming the Lake Monster':

> *'Now, when viewed from the surface, the inner reaches of the lake appeared as a kaleidoscope of color with a myriad of indescribably beautiful reflections. And so it was that the lake awoke and was no longer sad, since she now realized her own beauty. The sky and all of the animals were also able to see her magnificence, and they were especially happy since this reminded them of their own beauty, which they could clearly see reflected in her calm, still waters.'*

We Are All Creating The World

The 'butterfly effect' is a phrase coined by Edward Lorenz (mathematician, meteorologist and pioneer of 'chaos theory') which describes how every little action will create consequences that ripple outwards far afield:

> *'When a butterfly flaps its wings on one side of the earth, the effect may be felt on the other side of the world as a hurricane.'*

Since everything in life is part of a vast web of interconnectivity, the vibration of your energy field affects everything else throughout the Universe. Therefore, your karma doesn't only operate on a micro, 'personal' scale. With your expressions of compassion or selfishness, joy or suffering, peace or stress, and positive or negative viewpoint, you are, to a greater or lesser extent, helping to shape the world. So your positive vibration is extremely important for life. Howard Thurman expresses this eloquently:

> *'Don't ask what the world needs, ask what makes you come alive, and go do it. Because what the world needs is people who have come alive.'*

Since we're all creating the world, your vibration matters. When your lake monster is calm, your vibration will be contributing to love, peace, joy, unity, creativity and sustainability in the world. You really have no way of knowing just how far and wide your positive impact might be affecting life.

Was Arun's humility and positive frame of mind only felt by those in his village, or did he perhaps have an impact further afield? Maybe villagers from his village spoke of him with relatives in another village close by. His stature within the village might well have touched others whom he never met.

The way in which you positively or negatively impact upon life is determined by your inner vibration, which has little to do with your outward appearance or circumstances – clothes, cars, houses and bank accounts. It's your peace of mind and inner wellbeing which creates your positive influence.

So be careful not to 'judge a book by its cover'. The vastly contrasting perspectives in Chapter 1, 'The Predominant Trends Of Today', should not be judged superficially. It's quite possible that many of those people who 'appear' to have nothing are in fact far happier than those who appear to be successful, with their outer trappings of success that yield the 'superficial blip of calm and happiness'. Again, think of Arun.

You don't need to be rich to be happy; in fact, in many instances, the reverse is probably the case. Equally, you don't need to have much to give greatly. Giving of yourself is a quality of expressing yourself from the depth of your being, and therefore from a limitless well of creative energy. From here, abundance is the default setting, and love is the currency.

What is your predominant vibration?

Please consider this for a moment, because this is what you are giving to the world. It is so easy to look out at the world and see problems, disharmony, inequality and situations which just seem 'wrong'. But if you make your vibration one of non-acceptance, then this is what you project into the world, and you become a part of the problem.

There is great wisdom in the security announcement on a plane, which gives clear instructions to fit your own oxygen mask first before helping others with theirs. This is precisely what is meant by 'inner ecology before outer ecology', Satyananda's expression that I quoted at the beginning of the book. You can only contribute positively to a situation, or resolve a problem, by being in your *natural* frame of mind. From here, you will think, speak and act from a quality of mind that is imbued with universal wisdom and compassion. From here, you have the best chance to do whatever you can to resolve a situation:

You can only truly give to others once you yourself are well, not before

In most cases, your circle of influence is fairly limited in a direct sense. But, baring in mind the butterfly effect, you realize that your peace of mind is valuable to the rest of life.

Arun's family, and the local villagers who respected him so much, would not have known precisely the influence he had over their lives – but his impact was considerable for sure. I cannot begin to say what impact my dreams of flying have had on my life; but what I know for sure, is that they have played a significant role in this book. Perhaps my dreams of flying will therefore also touch others indirectly.

I would like to offer three examples of the Law of Magic (part 2), where individuals, or groups of individuals, have pursued their heartfelt desires, and this has greatly impacted upon the lives of others:

1. 'The Troubles'

In 1974, when I was 11 years old, my family participated in an initiative to bring children from Northern Ireland across to London, where they would stay in homes like ours, in the south-west of London.

The intention of the organizers was to bring together both Protestants and Catholics from Belfast, the epicenter of the conflict in Northern Ireland. At that time the conflict, which came to be known as 'The Troubles', was at its height. Violence on the streets of Northern Ireland was commonplace and spilled over into the Republic of Ireland and Great Britain.

Over the two weeks of providing a home to Clifford, we did our best to make him feel completely welcome. We never asked any direct questions about 'The Troubles', but it was clear to see that Clifford's life was overshadowed by great challenges.

At the end of the two weeks, on a Saturday evening in a church hall in Epsom, several miles outside of London, 50 Irish children and their temporary carers collected together for a party. The Irish children were mostly gathered in groups of five or six, all in the same area of the hall. What was beautiful to see was that there was no separation by religion. They were more like a single, vibrant huddle.

At a certain point, the DJ said over the microphone, 'Would all the children like to come on stage, I believe that they would like to sing for us.'

What happened next is so vivid in my memory, it's as though it had happened last week. Fifty Irish children began to sing a song that I had never heard before – 'When Irish Eyes Are Smiling'.

I believe that everyone in that room witnessed an event that night which left them awestruck. It was the combination of such passion for being Irish, coupled with the significance of their unity, rather than their differences, which so touched the hearts of all those who were present.

As a result of their heartfelt desire to create some unity amidst 'The Troubles', the organizers of this initiative deeply touched the lives of those 50 children. For sure, it was a transformational experience for them, and we have no way of knowing the effect that those two weeks, or that evening, had on the children's families and friends, or, indeed, their English hosts.

2. *Professor Stephen Hawking*

I spoke of Stephen Hawking earlier, in the context of the totality of wellbeing being so much more vast than merely the physical 'vehicle' which transports us around.

As I said before, he was first diagnosed with motor neuron disease when he was 21. At first, he was depressed and saw little point in continuing his studies at Cambridge. In fact, he was given just two years to live by the doctors. But he quickly accepted his predicament and remained, as he always had been, fiercely independent, and therefore unwilling to make concessions for his disabilities. In fact, he became renowned for his daredevil antics with his wheelchair, much as he had done a few years before, as a cox for his college rowing team at Cambridge.

He preferred to be regarded as 'a scientist first, popular science writer second, and, in all the ways that matter, a normal human being with the same desires, drives, dreams, and ambitions as the next person'. He has three children with his first wife Jane, and today, at the ripe old age of 74, Professor Hawking is held in the very highest regard as a mathematician, theoretical physicist, cosmologist and all-round genius, by peers, presidents and the common man alike.

He is such a marvelous example for us all, since he embodies the very essence of the Law of Magic. In spite of being wheelchair bound, and only able to speak by activating a single muscle in his cheek, he hasn't let this remotely diminish his passion for solving the greatest scientific challenges of our times. In so doing, he demonstrates beyond all doubt that when we pursue our heartfelt dreams, we are also serving humanity.

3. Narayanan Krishnan

> *'I saw a very old man he was eating his own human waste for hunger. I thought, what is the purpose of my life? ... In the Taj hotel I feed all my guests, but there in my home town there are people who are living even without food ...'*

So begins Narayan's TEDxTalk: 'The Joy Of Giving'.¹ At the tender age of 21, Narayan had a promising career as a chef with the Taj Hotel Group in Bangalore. He was about to be sent to Switzerland for a four-year placement, and so he called his mother to tell her his plans.

She asked him to come home for a few days, and do some pujas (prayers) in his local temple. It was during this trip that Narayanan saw the decrepit old man (whom he spoke about in the above quote) lying by the side of the street, as well as so many other starving, destitute people who were completely uncared for. This was a defining moment in his life, and Narayanan decided to quit his job, and take on the daunting task of feeding and caring for the starving, homeless people in his hometown of Madurai, Tamil Nadu, in India.

Using his own savings, Narayanan fed around 30 people to begin with. The next year, he started to serve freshly cooked meals, and, since then, up until August 2011, he had served over 1.7 million meals. But it wasn't just about feeding these homeless people, he also cut their hair, shaved them and bathed them. He realized that whilst food would nourish them physically, they also needed psychological care, in the form of a hand to hold and someone to speak with. What is all the more impressive is that Narayanan is a Brahmin (the highest caste of the Hindu faith), and therefore he was not supposed to mix with these 'untouchables', let alone feed, touch and show such depth of love for them. But as he says in the video:

'What is the ultimate purpose of life? It is to give.'

Narayanan's incredible story of love and compassion for his fellow human beings embodies the very essence of 'karma yoga' – to give of yourself selflessly. What is so beautiful about this particular story is that when you watch the video, you will see how humble and yet alive Narayanan is. The possibility to serve others in the way that he does feeds him deeply, providing him with an abundant source of gratitude. This is an extremely powerful message for all of us.

In all three of these examples, the main characters were neither seeking fame nor adulation. Their hearts were open, and their minds were quiet, and the positive impact that they had was therefore extremely powerful. We all have this possibility to come alive and share our positive vibration with the world.

**When your mind is quiet, and your heart is open,
your positive vibration is a force for good.**

Practical Exercise

Please answer the following questions. Before you begin, first SOAR.

- Can I remember a time recently (maybe right now), when I felt truly alive, and I could sense the positive impact that I was having on others?
- Can I see that my vibration is always impacting on those around me?

- Do I have any idea of how far my vibration might spread, and impact upon others?
- Do I have a sense of my part in the bigger picture of life?
- Does it inspire me to realize that being the best that I can be can help mankind?
- Can I begin to sense, if I hadn't already, that 'serving' others will truly fulfill me, and in a way that nothing else can?

Notes

1. Narayanan Krishnan, 'The Joy Of Giving: Narayanan Krishnan at TEDxGateway', YouTube, www.youtube.com/watch?v=-WPOEXZNEgg.

Summary Chapter 8

The Law of Magic (Part 2)
Your Coming Alive Serves Others

The Law of Magic (Part 2)

When you unleash your creative fire through pursuing what you truly desire, you come alive, and your positive vibration touches others. Coming alive is therefore your gift to the world.

Your Vibration Matters

No matter who you are, you can be inspired to come alive and allow your positive vibration to touch others.

We Are All Creating the World

According to the 'butterfly effect', every single action, whether fearful or loving, will create consequences that ripple outwards far afield. Your greatest gift to the world, therefore, is that you come alive, and transmit a positive vibration –

> *'Don't ask what the world needs, ask what makes you come alive, and go do it. Because what the world needs is people who have come alive.'*

In order to positively impact upon a situation, or the world in general, you first need to be relaxed and well yourself – in your *natural* frame of mind.

Chapter 9

SOARing

Being the Master of My Own Wellbeing

The intention of this chapter is to pull together all of the lessons of the book, and express them in one clear message:

Be the master of your own wellbeing and impact positively upon the rest of humanity by consistently inviting your *natural* quality of your mind.

This book has been written as a journey of three parts. The three parts provide you with three keys, and their corresponding tools, introduced in a particular order. This order is important, because even though the keys are inseparable, each supports the next.

- **1st Key: Learn To Calm Your Mind – 'Relax'** – Wake Up and SOAR
- **2nd Key: Take Charge of Your Wellbeing – 'Nurture'** – Your Personal Support System
- **3rd Key: Pursue Your Dreams – 'Fly'** – The Law of Magic

Part 1: The book begins by expressing the problem that humans face – the *normal* quality of mind. This creates the *normal* 'problem trends'. Yet, once you realize that you can control your quality of mind, you sense a great opportunity, which is to choose your *natural* quality of mind. Wake Up and SOAR is the tool that allows you to do this, so that you can relax at will.

The essence of SOAR is that you find peace with all that is arising within and outside of you. In other words, you embrace acceptance. So you neither attach to your thoughts, unless you truly want to, and nor do you resist them. The 10 Mantras are an additional tool which invites surrendered acceptance.

Part 2: When you know how to calm your mind, you're able to design your Personal Support System in such a way that it will truly nurture you – allowing you to optimize your health and happiness when you're well, and support your own healing when you're stressed or sick.

Part 3: When you feel nurtured and supported, you are able to come alive through pursuing your heartfelt desires and therefore fly without risk of stress or sickness:

- The Law of Magic (Part 1) shows you how to come alive, which will feed you deeply.

- The Law of Magic (Part 2) shows you that when you come alive this serves others too. Inspiring others and inviting them towards calmness is your gift to the world.

Your journey through the three parts of the book awakens you to the realization that you can truly love your life by creating a virtuous circle of inviting and surfing your *natural* quality of mind.

- Wake Up and SOAR – accesses your *natural* quality of mind
- Personal Support System – nurtures your *natural* quality of mind
- The Law of Magic – surfs your *natural* quality of mind

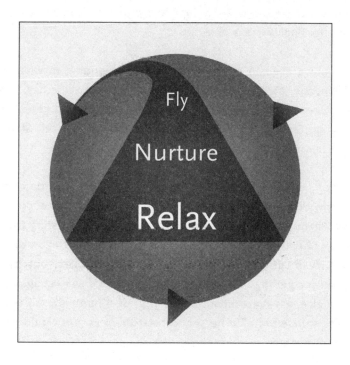

A virtuous circle of inviting your natural quality of mind

SOARing

Because many people tend to be predominantly in the *normal* state, experiencing varying forms and degrees of fear and uncertainty, this inevitably creates and perpetuates the 'problem trends'. Right now matters are perhaps more serious than ever before, because we wield such power to impact upon one another and our biosphere. If we don't alter our collective trajectory, we will find ourselves inhabiting a planet that is increasingly inhospitable.

As a race, we need to re-calibrate our understanding of what life is really all about. We can sugar-coat it, but at the end of the day, in spite of life's incredible beauty and magnificence, it can also be extremely challenging. So for me, real success in life, or what I call SOARing, could be described as:

Journeying beyond your story on the road less traveled, the one that points inwards, not outwards; meeting challenges head on whilst smiling as you walk towards your heartfelt dreams; trusting that you are being guided and taken care of through thick and thin; measuring your achievements not by kind words and accolades, but by your ability to keep getting back up after you've fallen down yet again; and, above all else, having compassion for your own humanity, so that you recognize yourself in all others, and treat them as you would wish to be treated yourself.

SOARing requires that you integrate the three keys into your life so that you are relaxed, you feel supported, and you are vibrantly alive. Ultimately, this means that you spend much of your time doing what you love to do. But it also means that you adjust the lens through which you perceive your life, so that what was perhaps previously unacceptable or undesirable is now seen as something that you wish to embrace, since it's an integral part of what you truly desire.

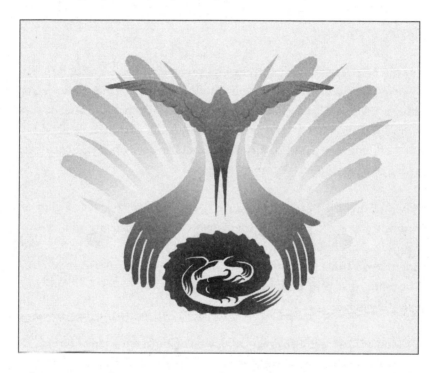

When you're relaxed (Wake Up and SOAR), and you feel nurtured (Personal Support System), you empower yourself to fly through pursuing your heartfelt desires and feeling vibrantly alive. This will bring you real joy and allow you to positively impact others (Law of Magic). When you realize that riding your magic carpet and pursuing your heartfelt desires not only feeds you deeply, but also benefits those around you, then you start to live your life from the perspective of service. In Indian philosophy, this is your dharma – your purpose. This will yield true and enduring fulfillment.

Giving of Yourself

Let me be clear about what I mean by service. When you recognize the symbiosis between what feeds you, and the way in which this also feeds others, there is no longer a separation between the two. Instead, you simply wish to humbly serve life. You realize that what is truly good for you – coming alive – is good for all, and your overriding purpose becomes giving of yourself through coming alive.

When taking good care of your own needs harmonizes with giving of yourself, there is a magical alchemy which arises, causing you to love your life. This is because you are designed to function as part of the one human tribe. It's not that you have to behave like everyone else, but rather that you recognize, at depth, your unity with everyone and everything else:

Mother Nature is a self-regulating web of life in a myriad of forms, where each element exists as part of the grand plan to maintain the health of the whole.

Perhaps you've already discovered that when your plans are egocentric, they don't really fulfill you. But when they emanate from the depth of your being, and embrace your wish to have a positive impact on those around you, or humanity as a whole, then you are supported by life and you feel truly fulfilled.

This includes the possibility for you to see the positive in someone who is behaving selfishly, or has hurt you in some way. Think of Malala in the first of the 10 Mantras – 'Be Positive and Open to Opportunities':

'At first I thought that I would hit him with a shoe. Then I thought if you hit a Talib with a shoe, then there would be no difference between you and the Talib ... You must not treat others with cruelty ... You must fight others through peace and through dialogue and through education.'

If you think that you've been betrayed, abandoned, manipulated or whatever it may be, can you find it in your heart to have compassion for the protagonist or protagonists, as Malala did? Can you see that they were perhaps utterly lost in a *normal* state of mind?

Not only will this serve you deeply, since your surrendered acceptance allows you to maintain peace of mind, but you will also create the space for the 'wrongdoer' to sense their wrongdoing, and perhaps wake up in the process.

Your coming alive serves others

There are many examples of loving souls who have walked the Earth throughout the course of history. Some of them, such as Buddha, Jesus, Mohammad, Gandhi, Nelson Mandela, Mother Theresa and so on, have profoundly impacted human history.

But there are countless other human beings, just like you and me, who manage to transcend life's profound programing and walk the road less traveled. Although their names are not recorded in history books, their influence touches those around them and causes a ripple of happiness to follow in their wake.

These people have found the strength to break free from the status quo of the *normal* state, and instead are acting more consistently from a higher, *natural* quality of mind – SOARing. This has nothing to do with their job or position, and they are just as likely to be bus drivers, office clerks, cleaners or athletes as they are spiritual leaders. Anyone can come alive and touch others with their positive vibration.

The most potent way to be happy and fulfilled is to give of yourself, like the organizers, and the Irish children up on stage, in the story about 'The Troubles'; like Stephen Hawking; and like Narayanan. As Albert Schweitzer said, 'The purpose of human life is to serve and to show compassion and the will to help others.' The incredible thing about giving selflessly, because this arises naturally within you, is that you inspire others to be the best that they can be.

So the key message that I stated at the start of this chapter, becomes:

Be the master of your own wellbeing and impact positively upon the rest of humanity through consistently inviting your *natural* quality of your mind. This will inspire others to come alive, and together we can positively transform the world.

Life is meant to flow, just like a river to the ocean; and that flow is from the inside out, not the other way around. From surrendered acceptance, and the resulting calmness, you will naturally take good care of yourself, and therefore pursue your dreams happily, in the knowledge that this is your gift to life. But before flying, make sure that you have a solid base, otherwise your ability to fly becomes your downfall. There are a myriad of examples of sad and depressed 'superstars', who didn't have the capacity to deal with the pursuit of their dreams and the resulting fame and fortune.

So if you truly want to help humanity, be aware of the energetic vibration that you are emitting, since everything is inextricably intertwined, and your every thought, word and action impact upon the rest of life. Your commitment to being fully alive and SOARing is therefore the key to awakening others to the same beautiful possibility.

In Conclusion

Your life experience, and every aspect of your wellbeing, begins with your quality of mind, and this begins with your predominant thoughts:

In the moment you realize that you are in some way resisting life by attaching to an unsolicited thought, or a disturbing emotion, and you choose to not continue that thought, or to not give attention to that emotion or sensation, you set yourself free.

Whatever you focus your mind on, you enliven it with your life force, and generate a vibration that is transmitted throughout your being, and out into the world. So if you continually believe that the programed thoughts and emotions which arise in your body-mind are who you are, then you attract, and gradually become, their likeness. As Buddha said:

'The mind is everything. What you think you become.'

Your wellbeing is about making the most of your compelling possibility rather than being the victim of your genetic programing and life's conditioning. You have the magical capacity to unleash your creative fire at will, so that you live in the *natural* realm of magic, and not the *normal* realm of projecting a conditioned story onto the screen of life. When you engage the Law of Magic fully, you learn to love your life through constantly opening your heart and mind.

If you have been responding to my prompts and suggestions, and completing the practical exercises along the way, then you will already be well on your way to integrating the three keys into your life. My suggestion is that you regularly re-read the book, particularly those sections which you've highlighted, or which have touched you the most.

But also, you might be pleased to hear that our interaction doesn't have to finish with the book — at least not from my perspective. Please read on ...

What Next?

Perhaps you remember what I said in the introduction about the 'hot bath effect' – that it is often hard to remain inspired and committed to the cause, once you've 'climbed out of the bath'. In other words, in the context of this book, the real test begins when you put the book down, having read the last words of the last page.

As I have said a few times, I believe that in today's world we would all benefit greatly from some form of 'support system'. By this I am referring to something that is in addition to a loving family, a supportive group of friends, and the 'three keys'. Perhaps this book has moved you in some way, and I sincerely hope that it has. But what if it fed into an ongoing possibility for guidance and support?

I have mentioned the idea of co-creating a wellbeing portal, and how this might empower and support you in taking responsibility for your wellbeing, as well as act as a validating force for the holistic and natural healthcare realm – HNH. My team and I are therefore delighted to be able to give you the link to the following site, which gives details of our SOAR app:

www.soar-app.com

The vision for the SOAR app grew from creating and running the Ashiyana Retreat Village. Our experiences over the last ten years have given us a deep insight into both the pressures of modern-day living, and the support and guidance required for a return to balance.

Our long-term vision for the app, is therefore to create a comprehensive support system, based on the three keys. But to begin with, the app will be focused on enabling you to find a wellbeing practitioner in your area – it will geolocate you and then allow you to book a practitioner who will visit you at your home or office.

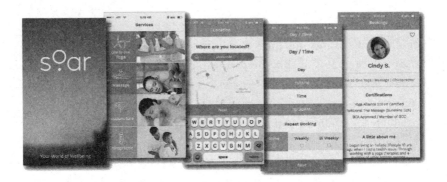

For every transaction that happens through the app, we will give £1 to one of the causes that we are supporting – 'Giving'. (Right now, these are the 'Nepal Project' that I've mentioned a couple of times, the Satsang Foundation which supports Satyananda's work, and the 'Alto Project' in Brazil – a bioforestry project which also supports those struggling with addiction in the local town.)

In the future, we will offer members the possibility to share information and ideas freely. We intend to become a platform for supporting and promoting what works in the world of holistic and natural healthcare (HNH), as well as offering a breadth of validated information, guidance and inspiration.

Our app will become the first one-stop, global wellbeing platform, designed to facilitate wellbeing, create loving community and raise consciousness.

If you feel that you would like to, please download the app, and if you're pleased with what you see and experience, then invite like-minded friends to download it as well. The sooner we have a critical mass of members, the faster we will be able to add to the functionality and offer you a comprehensive, global, wellbeing platform.

For more information about Ashiyana, me, 'Giving' and this and other books, please check – www.wakeupandsoar.com

My contact details – chris@wakeupandsoar.com

Satyananda's contact details – www.satyananda.org

Namaste

'My soul honors your soul. I honor the place in you in which the entire Universe resides. I honor the place in you which is of love, of light, of truth, of beauty and of peace. When you are in that place in you, and I am in that place in me, We are United. We are the Same. We are One.'

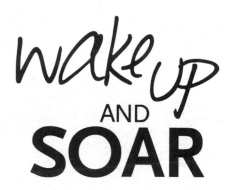